Diabetic Foot - Recent Advances

Edited by Alok Raghav

Published in London, United Kingdom

Diabetic Foot - Recent Advances
http://dx.doi.org/10.5772/intechopen.102211
Edited by Alok Raghav

Contributors
Wakuma Wakene Jifar, Steven Coon, Saminathan Jayapal, Nandu Bhavani Murugesan, Sasikala Mohan, James Monroe Laborde, Lingyan Zhu, Yu Xiao, Yao Xiao, Yinan Jiang, Maharana Prathap Reddy Adama, George K. Gittes, Manoharlal Manoj Abraham, Subramaniam Hari Hara Sudan, Venugopal Pavithra, Nataraj Nithya, Pradhapsankar Veeramani, Suganya Murugeshan, Idris Long, Faiz Ahmed Shaikh, Muhammad Ilyas Nadeem, Deephikaa Ramakrishnan Ramesh, George J. Dugbartey, Karl K. Alornyo

First published in London, United Kingdom, 2023 by IntechOpen
IntechOpen is the global imprint of INTECHOPEN LIMITED, registered in England and Wales, registration number: 11086078, 5 Princes Gate Court, London, SW7 2QJ, United Kingdom

British Library Cataloguing-in-Publication Data
A catalogue record for this book is available from the British Library

Additional hard and PDF copies can be obtained from orders@intechopen.com

Diabetic Foot - Recent Advances
Edited by Alok Raghav
p. cm.
Print ISBN 978-1-83880-814-3
Online ISBN 978-1-83880-815-0
eBook (PDF) ISBN 978-1-83880-816-7

Meet the editor

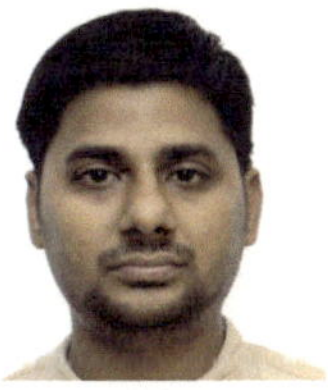

Dr. Alok Raghav obtained his Ph.D. in Endocrinology from Rajiv Gandhi Centre for Diabetes and Endocrinology, J.N. Medical College, Faculty of Medicine, Aligarh Muslim University, India. He worked as a project scientist at the Indian Institute of Technology in Kanpur, India. He has more than ten years of research experience in the field of glycobiology and diabetes mellitus. He also worked as Scientist C at the Multidisciplinary Research Unit (sponsored by the Department of Health Research, Ministry of Health and Family Welfare, New Delhi), GSVM Medical College Kanpur, India. He is currently working as a Research Professor at the School of Medicine, Department of Anatomy & Cell Biology, Lee Gil Ya Cancer and Diabetes Institute, Gachon University, South Korea. Dr. Raghav has received several international and national awards. He is also an associate editor for *Frontiers in Endocrinology and Frontiers in Public Health* and an academic editor for *PLOS One.*

Contents

Preface

Diabetic foot ulcers (DFUs) are a secondary complication of diabetes mellitus. This book provides a comprehensive overview of DFUs with chapters that reflect the wide range of research currently being practiced in the field.

The book is organized into three sections on pathophysiology, treatment, and assessment. It begins with an introductory chapter that provides an overview of DFUs. Subsequent chapters discuss options for effective management and treatment of this complication. Advances in medical science have led to the development of novel treatments for DFUs, including point-of-care devices for home use.

The link between diabetic foot ulcers and an increased risk of amputation, morbidity, and mortality is well documented in the literature, including guidelines from several international organizations. Thus, proper management and care of patients with DFUs may help to reduce healthcare burdens and associated costs.

We would like to thank the authors for their excellent contributions. We would also like to acknowledge Author Service Manager Ms. Maja Bozicevic at IntechOpen for her assistance throughout the publication process.

Alok Raghav
Research Professor,
School of Medicine,
Department of Anatomy and Cell Biology,
Gachon University,
Incheon, South Korea

Section 1

Pathophysiology

Chapter 1

Association between Diabetic Kidney Disease and Diabetic Foot Ulceration

George J. Dugbartey and Karl K. Alornyo

Abstract

Diabetic kidney disease (DKD) is a common global health challenge characterized by a decline in renal function among the diabetic population, which progresses to end-stage renal disease (ESRD). Evidence in the literature suggests a strong association between DKD and the development of diabetic foot ulceration (DFU). DFU is a serious health issue that complicates both type 1 and type 2 diabetes mellitus, and negatively impacts the quality of life of diabetic patients. Patients with advanced DKD or ESRD have a five-fold increased risk of developing DFU, with 6.5–10 times higher rate of amputation than their non-nephropathic counterparts. Multiple and inter-related pathways of DFU in DKD have been identified in which ischemia, neuropathy and infection are major contributing pathologies. However, extensive research to comprehensively assess the progression of DFU in DKD is lacking. In this chapter, we discuss the causal pathways in DFU development and progression, the relationship between DKD and DFU as well as treatment options and measures to achieve both primary and secondary prevention.

Keywords: diabetic kidney disease (DKD), diabetic foot ulceration (DFU), end-stage renal disease (ESRD), chronic kidney disease (CKD), diabetes mellitus, amputation

1. Introduction

Diabetic foot ulceration (DFU) is a serious complication of diabetes mellitus worldwide, and the most common cause of in-patient admissions among the diabetic population [1, 2]. It reduces mobility and quality of life of patients. Left untreated or poorly managed, DFU can lead to amputation, and death in extreme cases [3]. The etiology of DFU is quite complex due to the involvement of a number of pathophysiological mechanisms, with polyneuropathy being the most crucial of them all [4, 5]. Proper adherence to standard treatment strategies (both pharmacological and non-pharmacological) and interdisciplinary cooperation between healthcare practitioners (doctors, nurses, pharmacists, etc.) and the patient can reduce the relatively high rates of major amputations and mortality in diabetic patients due to DFU [6–8].

Diabetes-related foot complications have been identified as the most common cause of morbidity among diabetic patients [1]. Peripheral vascular disease is a major underlying risk factor for the development of DFU due to reduced oxygenation of the foot. It renders the diabetic foot asymptomatic until latter evidence of non-healing ulcers become evident [9, 10]. Also, uremia due to diabetic kidney disease (DKD) reduces the body's immune capabilities and creates a suitable environment for bacterial growth in the foot ulcers [11]. Inadequate oxygenation or perfusion of the affected foot aids in the progression of DFU due to a reduced delivery of antibiotics to the affected foot. At this point, the patient needs to be monitored strictly to prevent the steady progression of DFU to diabetic gangrene, a condition where foot ulcerations become necrotic and unresponsive to antibiotic therapy and ultimately may require amputation of the affected foot [12, 13].

While about 6.3% of patients currently have foot ulcerations worldwide [14], it is estimated that about 25% of diabetic patients may develop DFU in their lifetime [5]. Of all amputations in diabetic patients, 85% are preceded by DFU, which subsequently worsens to a gangrene or infection [3, 15]. DFU is more prevalent in type 2 diabetic patients, with these patients suffering recurring hospital admissions which increases their financial burden on the healthcare system and the patient [16]. Everett and Mathioudakis [17] recently reported that diabetic patients with DFU have 2.5 times increase of dying while experiencing an 11-fold increase in hospital costs compared to patients hospitalized for nondiabetic foot ulcer. A patient's likelihood of developing DFU increases as his or her disease duration increases [18], while complications such as DKD further increases the patient's risk of getting foot ulcers [19]. Furthermore, the severity of DFU delays wound healing time [18, 20], which consequently increases the cost of its clinical management. This chapter discusses the causal pathways in DFU development and progression, the relationship between DKD and DFU as well as treatment options and measures to achieve both primary and secondary prevention.

2. Pathophysiology of diabetic foot ulceration

DFU is a complex condition which has a host of pathological mechanisms involved in its development and progression. Thus, multiple and inter-related pathways of DFU have been identified in which diabetic peripheral neuropathy, peripheral vascular disease and ischemia, and infection are major contributing pathologies [21–23].

2.1 Diabetic peripheral neuropathy

Diabetic peripheral neuropathy (DPN) is considered the cardinal driving force to developing DFU. It is a condition where nerves in the limbs (lower limbs in the case of DFU) are damaged by a variety of conditions such as inflammation, oxidative stress, advanced glycated end-products and a decrease in nitric oxide production [24–26]. The nerve damage renders the diabetic feet insensitive to harmful stimuli such as trauma from stepping on a hot or sharp object or skin injury from wearing ill-fitted shoes. It is reported that over 60% of foot ulcers among the diabetic population is directly linked to the development of DPN [24–26]. An increased activity of aldose reductase and sorbitol dehydrogenase (enzymes involved in the alternate metabolism of glucose under hyperglycemic conditions) leads to the accumulation of sorbitol and fructose [27]. High concentrations of these sugars negatively impact the levels of myoinositol, a carbocyclic sugar that mediates cell signal transduction in response to neurotransmitter and hormones [28, 29]. In DPN, there is reduced nerve innervation of small muscles of the foot as well as a decline in peripheral sensation and vasomotor control of the pedal circulation. This leads to development of wounds in these patients, which progress to ulcers that go unnoticed until observed by someone else [30].

Diabetes mellitus also promotes skin fissuring and dryness (reduced sweating), a situation which makes the skin prone to infections (due to the cracks in the skin acting as a potential portal for entry of bacteria) and poses as a risk factor in the expansion and worsening of DFU [31, 32].

DPN may reduce the production of neuropeptides such as substance P, calcitonin gene-related peptide and nerve growth factor, as these neuropeptides are important for wound healing [33–35]. These changes aid the progression of wounds and ulcers to gangrenes, coupled untimely management (with pharmacological or surgical intervention) ultimately leads to the loss of a limb. Also, the lack of pain sensation exposes the feet of diabetic patients with sensory neuropathy to repeated unnoticed trauma. It is important to note that the lack of pain sensation and impaired temperature sensation, both being components of sensory neuropathy, can make the instant withdrawal of a foot from harmful objects or hot liquid impossible [36, 37]. This creates an ulcer which may become chronic due to constant exposure to obnoxious stimuli. Furthermore, repeated pressure at focal point within the foot leads to the development of foot ulcers. This is partly linked to flexor extension imbalance and muscle atrophy, which develops in some diabetic patients, causing unequal distribution pressure and prominence of the diabetic foot [38, 39]. Thus, DPN creates repeated and unequal distribution pressure in the feet of diabetic patients, leading to development of DFU.

2.2 Peripheral vascular disease and ischemia

Hypoperfusion (ischemia) resulting from peripheral vascular disease contributes to DFU development due to reduced oxygen supply to the diabetic foot [40]. The vascular disease in diabetic patients is mostly localized in arteries of the lower limb, with dismal prognosis [41, 42]. A major risk factor for the development of peripheral vascular disease is atherosclerosis [43, 44], a condition in which an artery become hardened or thickened due to a buildup of plaque in its inner lining. Atherosclerosis appears at a younger age in diabetic individuals and progresses more rapidly than in nondiabetic individuals [45, 46], thus making diabetes mellitus one of the risk factors for developing atherosclerosis. In the diabetic microcirculation, there is existence of structural changes, most notably, a thickening of the capillary basement membrane and endothelial dysfunction [47, 48]. As already mentioned, DPN reduces the production of neuropeptides which aid in wound healing [33–35]. These neuropeptides directly and indirectly (through mast cell release of histamine) cause increased permeability and vasodilation [49, 50]. The endothelium plays an important role in blood vessel wall function by synthesizing and releasing vasodilators such as prostaglandins and nitric oxide, which modulate vascular tone in pedal circulation [51, 52]. A host of mechanisms responsible for vascular dysfunction in diabetes have been identified to include over-production of reactive oxygen species, impaired nitric oxide pathway, abnormal production of vasoconstrictor prostanoids, intracellular signaling and advanced glycated end products [53–55]. This pathological vascular alteration in the diabetic foot contributes to DFU development, suggesting that diabetic patients must undergo a timely vascular examination for timely revascularization.

2.3 Infection

The immune system of healthy people is much more robust and stronger than that of diabetic individuals [56, 57] and thus, foot infections in the latter group need to be closely monitored and managed appropriately [58, 59]. Unsurprisingly, it is estimated that about 50% of patients with DFU present clinical signs of infection (either locally or systemically) [60, 61]. A foot infection is characterized by the presence of purulent secretions or at least two of the classic signs of inflammation (erythema, hyperemia, edema, or swelling and pain) [62, 63]. Patients with poor metabolic or uncontrolled diabetes are commonly afflicted with bacterial infection in which a lack of granulation tissue, delayed healing, appearance of necrotic tissue on wound surface and/or odor are prominent [64, 65]. Furthermore, these patients display a loss of sensitivity (i.e. diabetic peripheral neuropathy) in the affected foot due to damage caused to short and long fibers (A-beta and A-delta) secondary to hyperglycemia [66, 67]. Chronic hyperglycemia, a hallmark of diabetes mellitus, provides a suitable medium for bacterial growth, mainly aerobic Gram-positive cocci (e.g. *Staphylococcus aureus*), Gram-negative aerobes (e.g. *Pseudomonas aeruginosa*) and drug-resistant bacteria such as vancomycin-resistant *S. aureus* and methicillin-resistant *S. aureus*, which were the common microorganisms identified in the diabetic foot [68–70]. In extreme situations, the bacterial infection of soft tissue spreads to the bones (causing osteomyelitis; an inflammation in the bone) and other surrounding tissues and organs. Unsuccessful attempts at halting the spread of the infection may lead to septicemia and amputation of the affected limb [65, 70]. Also, uncontrolled diabetes mellitus impairs the proliferation of fibroblasts and collagen synthesis while prolonging an inflammatory cascade [71, 72], a condition which compromises the wound healing abilities of diabetic patients. In summary, persistent hyperglycemia in diabetic individuals creates a suitable microenvironment for the growth of pathogenic bacteria, which contributes to DFU development and progression.

3. Renal involvement in diabetic foot ulceration

3.1 Diabetic patients with chronic kidney disease and end-stage renal disease

Chronic kidney disease (CKD) is clinically defined by the presence of persistent albuminuria (albumin-to-creatinine ratio ≥ 30 mg/g for at least 3 months) regardless of etiology [73, 74]. It is estimated that about 40% of patients with DKD are expected to develop CKD at a point in their life [75]. The progression of CKD to end-stage renal disease (ESRD; the final stage of CKD) is higher in diabetic patients compared to their nondiabetic counterpart, so as is the mortality rate of these patients with DFU [76]. Calciphylaxis, uremic pruritus and nephrogenic systemic fibrosis are skin disorders that increase the risk of DFU development in patients with DKD [77–79]. Calciphylaxis, for example, presents with painful skin lesions which progress into a necrotic nonhealing skin ulcer and occasionally, gangrene in ESRD patients. It is a rare and life-threatening complication in which calcium accumulates in small blood vessels of the skin, occurring in about 1% of ESRD patients annually [78, 80]. Although its exact pathophysiology remains unclear, some studies suggest that abnormal bone and mineral metabolism, hyperparathyroidism, and vitamin D therapy contribute to the development of this disorder [81, 82]. Given that the most common clinical presentation of calciphylaxis is nonhealing lower extremity ulcers, its timely identification by relevant healthcare professionals is critical [83, 84].

As diabetic peripheral neuropathy is one of the major contributing factors in DFU development and progression, uremic neuropathy, a sensorimotor neuropathy caused by uremic toxins, is a common complication of ESRD in which glomerular filtration rate (GFR) of the patient is <12 mL/min due to a buildup of dialyzable neurotoxins [85, 86]. The coexistence of uremic neuropathy and diabetes mellitus suggests that the clinical manifestations of diabetic neuropathy overlap with uremic neuropathy in diabetic patients with CKD and/or ESRD. Diabetic patients with ESRD also show immune vulnerability to infections, as hyperglycemia creates a veritable medium for bacterial growth and infection. As such, infections account for the second cause of mortality next to cardiovascular etiologies among diabetic patients with ESRD, representing 20% of the death of these patients, and also contributes significantly to their morbidity partly due to a decreased bactericidal activity of neutrophils [87, 88]. Moreover, pathological changes in complement function and significantly elevated levels of pro-inflammatory cytokines were associated with reduced renal clearance and persistent infection in diabetic patients with ESRD [89, 90].

In addition to uremic neuropathy and infection in diabetic patients, peripheral vascular disease was also found to increase the progression and severity of DFU, with an incidence rate in patients with CKD stage 1, 2 and 3 or 4 to be 4.7, 4.9 and 8.6 respectively [91, 92]. Of note, the risk factors for DFU can be seen in all stages of CKD, with microalbuminuria (the major clinical feature of DKD) as an independent risk factor for DFU [93]. Interestingly, Margolis et al. [94] found that the hazards of DFU increased by twofold and threefold in patients with CKD stage 3 and 4 respectively, while the risk for DFU decreased with improvement in renal function. ESRD, the final stage of CKD, increases the frequency of DFU and other foot complications such as infection, gangrene and amputation, with a twofold increase in diabetic patients relative to their non-ESRD counterparts [95, 96]. A previous study involving a cross-sectional examination of diabetic patients with and without ESRD also showed a fourfold increased risk of DFU complication among those with ESRD compared to their non-nephropathic diabetic counterparts [95]. These reports were later supported by the findings of Wolf and colleagues [97], who also observed that every 10 mL/min increase in estimated GFR (eGFR; a test of renal function and stage of CKD) corresponded with a 30% and 13% decrease in the odds of developing DFU in type 1 and type 2 diabetic patients respectively. As ESRD is associated with increase in diabetic foot complications such as amputation, a substantial body of evidence shows that amputation rate among diabetic patients with ESRD is 6.5–10 times higher compared to non-nephropathic diabetic population [96, 98, 99], with a low chance of diabetic wound healing as well as failure of healing from transmetatarsal amputations [100–105]. Also, a retrospective study of the effect of renal function on the development, severity, and outcome of DFU shows that reduced creatinine clearance increases the risk for DFU, with peripheral neuropathy and peripheral vascular disease also associated with DFU development [100].

Worsening the situation in diabetic patients with ESRD is the fact that tissue oxygenation is reduced as a result of decreased synthesis and release of erythropoietin (a hormone of renal origin which stimulates red blood cell production), culminating in anemia of ESRD, and thereby impairing diabetic wound healing [106–110]. Also, iron replacement therapy used by ESRD patients in the management of anemia has been recently shown to delay wound healing in these patients

[111]. This is because iron inhibits cofactor p300, needed for the synthesis and release of vascular endothelial growth factor (VEGF) by hypoxia inducible growth factor-1α [111]. VEGF regulates and maintains angiogenesis (a physiological process through which new blood vessels form from pre-existing vessels) [112, 113]. Results from recent preclinical studies suggest that iron depletion with deferoxamine (a heavy metal chelator) in rats improves tissue oxygenation and facilitates wound healing by curtailing iron-mediated impairment of VEGF upregulation [114]. Taken together, these findings imply that the range of DKD from microalbuminuria to ESRD represent a chain of risk factors for DFU development and progression.

3.2 Diabetic patients on renal dialysis

Another group of diabetic patients in which the kidney contributes to DFU development or progression are those receiving dialysis therapy. Dialysis patients who have markedly higher risks of DFU or amputation include those with previous foot ulceration or amputation, diabetes mellitus, DPN, or macrovascular disease [115, 116]. Other studies also found that reduced mobility and dexterity due to dialysis may impair the patient's ability to perform foot inspection or foot self-care. In addition, prolonged periods of inactivity on a dialysis couch for at least three times in a week could further contribute or worsen DFU by enhancing the development of pressure ulcers (prolonged pressure-induced skin injury) [117]. A retrospective study of 90 diabetic patients on dialysis therapy showed a high incidence of DFU and amputation before the start of dialysis, with a further increase following 2 years after dialysis initiation [115]. Therefore, it can be inferred that the dialysis treatment was a driving force in DFU progression and its complications. Such a negative effect of dialysis on DFU was later supported by the findings from a multiethnic study in which 400 diabetic patients on dialysis were reported to be at high risk for foot complications [118]. This finding was confirmed in another study by the same authors in which dialysis independently increased the risk for DFU in 137 diabetic patients, with an odd ration of 4.2 after including diabetic neuropathy, peripheral vascular disease, foot self-care measures and other potential confounders [119]. Miyajima et al. [102] also observed that major amputation rates are markedly increased in diabetic patients undergoing hemodialysis, with dismal prognosis while only half of diabetic patients on dialysis avoided major amputation regardless of revascularization [103]. In another study, amputation rate was reported to be 57% among diabetic patients receiving hemodialysis while 25% was reported in their counterparts with pre-dialysis ESRD [96]. In the same vein, diabetic patients on dialysis with critical foot ischemia had 8.9 times increased risk of poor prognosis [120].

McGrath and associate [121] also studied a close relationship between the time of dialysis initiation and development of diabetic foot complications. In a majority of diabetic patients, they found that the period from commencement of dialysis to amputation was less than 1 year, with the median being 7 months. Their observation was later corroborated by the findings of Game et al. [115] who reported a significant increase in the rate DFU onset by 3.3 (95% CI, 1.59–7.04) in the first year after commencement of dialysis while that between the second and fifth years increased by 4.56 (95% CI, 2.19–9.50). In the same study, the authors further reported that the increases in the incidence of major amputation were 31.98 (95% CI, 2.09–490.3) and 34.01 (95% CI, 1.74–666.2) in the first year and second to fifty year of dialysis respectively [115]. Similarly, compared to the general diabetic population, a 10-times increase in nontraumatic amputation rate was reported, as seen in 11.8–13.8/100 person-years in diabetic patients on dialysis [98], while diabetes mellitus was identified as the main risk factor for amputation of lower limb among patients on hemodialysis [122]. Tragically, the rates of mortality among amputees receiving dialysis therapy are disproportionately high regardless of successful post-amputation rehabilitation. For example, 50% mortality was reported within 1 year in 14 diabetic patients receiving dialysis therapy compared to 33% 1-year mortality rate in diabetic patients receiving treatment for heart failure [123]. Also, a study involving a large cohort of diabetic patients revealed increased post-amputation mortality rates, which corresponded with worsening renal condition, with dialysis patients being the most affected [124]. As infection (or sepsis) is a principal aggravating factor in DFU development and progression, it has been identified as a contributing factor next to cardiovascular disease in the mortality of diabetic patients on dialysis. A case-control study that sought to investigate the rates of mortality following diabetes-associated amputation revealed sepsis as a major cause of post-amputation mortality (49% of cases) compared to mortality due to heart-related diseases (45%) [125]. Although the authors did not include diabetic patients receiving dialysis therapy in their study, the implication of their findings is very important, as diabetic patients receiving dialysis treatment are easily vulnerable to infection. On a whole, dialysis increases the rate of DFU onset and progression as well as lower limb amputation and post-amputation mortality.

3.3 Renal transplantation in diabetic patients

There is limited data to the contribution of kidney transplantation on the onset and progression of DFU. However, it is well-known that as a result of induction and maintenance of immunosuppression in kidney transplant recipients, they represent a special group that is highly susceptible to infection. Diabetic patients in this group may develop DFU from opportunistic infections which require hospital admissions because these infections are difficult to treat. Moreover, their compromised immune system due to immunosuppressive therapy may impair wound healing. Such a condition may lead to septicemia which can progress to sepsis [126]. There are studies showing amputation rates as high as 30% in this group of patients [126–128]. It is important to note that peripheral vascular disease is common among renal transplant recipients [127, 129], which increases their risk for DFU development. In the light of this, Sharma et al. [130] recently reported that about 1 in 7 patients develop a new onset DFU following kidney transplantation or simultaneous pancreas-kidney transplantation although glycemic status is well-controlled. They also observed that DFU increases the risk of failure of the renal graft [130]. Although data regarding the effect of kidney transplantation on DFU development and progression are scarce, the few studies done so far suggest that kidney transplantation increases the risk of developing DFU.

4. Current treatment options and prevention

The management of DFU involves pharmacological, non-pharmacological approaches and/or surgery. A patient's suitability for each management option depends on factors such as state of the wound (non-infected, necrotic or gangrenous), required frequency for assessment, and the likelihood for patient compliance (mobility and financial capabilities).

4.1 Pharmacological approach

The selection of appropriate treatments should be based on the results of a wound culture once an infection is suspected. For accurate results during wound culture, it is ideal to harness tissue from the base of the ulcer after debridement rather than taken from a superficial wound [131, 132]. If deep tissue infections are suspected, specimens obtained aseptically during surgery provide optimal results. Chronic or previously treated wounds most often show polymicrobial growth, including Gram-positive cocci, Gram-negative rods or anaerobes and fungi in some cases [133]. Antibiotic-resistant organisms such as vancomycin-resistant *S. aureus* and methicillin-resistant *S. aureus* are frequently found in patients previously treated with antibiotic therapy or patients with a recent history of hospitalization or residence in a long-term care facility [134, 135]. The selection of appropriate antimicrobial therapy, including the agent, route of administration, and need for inpatient or outpatient treatment will be determined in part by the severity of the infection. In-patient admissions should be offered to individuals with systemic signs of severe infection with the provision of supportive care and intravenous antibiotic therapy based on result obtained from wound culture [136, 137]. Common classes of pharmacological agents used include lincosamides, fluoroquinolones, β-lactams/β-lactamase inhibitors [138, 139], and exogenous sources of agents such as nitric oxide that stimulate angiogenesis and vasodilation.

4.2 Non-pharmacological approach

4.2.1 Debridement

Debridement is one of the cornerstones of wound management, which could be surgical or non-surgical. It involves removal of necrotic tissue to aid wound healing. Debridement of open foot ulcers is required if unhealthy tissue is present, as this will aid in decreasing pressure points at callused sites on the foot [140, 141]. Removal of unhealthy tissue is linked to reducing colonizing a "clean" wound and allowing for examination of deep-lying tissues in the ulcer. Wound dressing is the cornerstone in diabetic foot care. As a convention, dressing changes and wound inspection and dressing should be done daily or as determined by the physician [142]. An ideal dressing should contribute to a moist wound environment, absorb excessive exudates, and not increase the risk for infections. Luckily, some non-surgical debriding agents have been incorporated with biologics such as transforming growth factor-β, vascular endothelial growth factor and epidermal growth factor [142–144]. Compared to conventional wound dressings, this modern wound dressing technique hastens the process of wound healing, as it stimulates angiogenesis, fibroblast proliferation, collagen synthesis and deposition, epithelization and remodeling of new extracellular matrix.

4.2.2 Surgery

Surgical management is considered an integral part of diabetic foot care, which is based on recent advances in technology and comprehensive understanding of the pathophysiology underlying DFU. Bypass surgery is a common method of treatment for ischemic limbs to preserve the functional anatomy of the diabetic foot. In cases where there are multiple levels of occlusion, surgery allows revascularization to restore arterial blood flow and increase the chance for limb salvage [145]. Prior to surgery, the possibility of underlying osteomyelitis should be considered with the presence of exposed bone [146]. The patient may undergo surgical excision of the affected bone or an extensive course of antibiotic therapy if septicemia is suspected [147].

4.3 Prevention of diabetic foot ulceration in patients with diabetic kidney disease

As DFU and its complications in patients with DKD either pre-, intra- or post-dialysis increases morbidity, mortality and financial burden, its prevention has become imperative. Unfortunately, foot care or chiropody programs have not been established in dialysis centers globally. This is a worrying picture, especially among patients with the highest risk of developing DFU. This group of patients include dialysis patients, amputees and those with history of foot ulceration. Emerging evidence shows that establishment of chiropody programs at dialysis units presents several benefits such as significant drop in the incidence of DFU among amputees and dialysis patients as well as reduction in the incidence of amputations, and improvement in ulcer healing times in the period when education on foot care and assessment, and provision of therapeutic shoes were introduced [148–151]. The beneficial outcomes of these preliminary studies suggest that instituting chiropody programs at all dialysis centers led by dialysis nurses would greatly reduce the burden of DFU and its complications on dialysis patients, healthcare system and society.

5. Conclusion

DFU is a common complication in diabetic patients, and remains a major cause of morbidity in patients with DKD. It has a complex pathophysiology involving a host of metabolic and hemodynamic processes such as diabetic peripheral neuropathy, ischemia (due to diabetic vascular disease) and infections. DFU deteriorates into gangrenes and necrotic wounds when left untreated or when not adequately attended to. Due to its complexity, a team of healthcare professionals are needed in the management of foot ulcerations involving both pharmacological and non-pharmacological interventions to address all three contributing pathologies (neuropathy, ischemia and infection). In some extraordinary cases, surgery maybe needed to provide revascularization, off-loading to relieve high-pressure areas and ultimately relief to patients. As there is significant renal contribution to DFU development and progression, preventive measures should include the need to institute chiropody programs at all dialysis centers to reduce the burden of DFU on dialysis patients, healthcare system and society.

Author details

George J. Dugbartey* and Karl K. Alornyo
Department of Pharmacology and Toxicology, School of Pharmacy, College of Health Sciences, University of Ghana, Accra, Ghana

*Address all correspondence to: gjdugbartey@ug.edu.gh; profduu@yahoo.com

References

[1] Lin C-W, Armstrong DG, Lin C-H, Liu P-H, Hung S-Y, Lee S-R, et al. Nationwide trends in the epidemiology of diabetic foot complications and lower-extremity amputation over an 8-year period. BMJ Open Diabetes Research & Care. 2019;**7**(1):1-7. DOI: 10.1136/bmjdrc-2019-000795

[2] Apelqvist J. The diabetic foot syndrome today: A pandemic uprise. Frontiers in Diabetes. 2018;**26**:1-18. DOI: 10.1159/000480040

[3] Zhang P, Lu J, Jing Y, Tang S, Zhu D, Bi Y. Global epidemiology of diabetic foot ulceration: A systematic review and meta-analysis. Annals of Medicine. 2017;**49**(2):106-116. DOI: 10.1080/07853890.2016.1231932

[4] Rastogi A, Goyal G, Kesavan R, Bal A, Kumar H, Mangalanadanam KP, et al. Long term outcomes after incident diabetic foot ulcer: Multicenter large cohort prospective study (EDI-FOCUS investigators) epidemiology of diabetic foot complications study. Diabetes Research and Clinical Practice. 2020;**162**:108113. DOI: 10.1016/j.diabres.2020.108113

[5] Ndip A, Ebah L, Mbako A. Neuropathic diabetic foot ulcers; evidence-to-practice. International Journal of General Medicine. 2012;**5**:129-134. DOI: 10.2147/IJGM.S10328

[6] Tuglo LS, Nyande FK, Agordoh PD, Nartey EB, Pan Z, Logosu L, et al. Knowledge and practice of diabetic foot care and the prevalence of diabetic foot ulcers among diabetic patients of selected hospitals in the Volta Region, Ghana. International Wound Journal. 2022;**19**(3):601-614. DOI: 10.1111/iwj.13656

[7] Kuguyo O, Muhaso C, Nyandoro S, Chirenda J, Chikwasha V, Mageza AC, et al. Perspectives of healthcare workers on factors influencing diabetes management and diabetic foot problems in Zimbabwe. JEMDSA. 2020;**25**(3):57-62. DOI: 10.1080/16089677.2020.1817283

[8] Rubio JA, Jiménez S, Lázaro-Martínez JL. Mortality in patients with diabetic foot ulcers: Causes, risk factors, and their association with evolution and severity of ulcer. Journal of Clinical Medicine. 2020;**9**(9):1-14. DOI: 10.3390/jcm9093009

[9] Brownrigg JRW, Apelqvist J, Bakker K, Schaper NC, Hinchliffe RJ. Evidence-based management of PAD & the diabetic foot. European Journal of Vascular and Endovascular Surgery. 2013;**45**(6):673-681. DOI: 10.1016/j.ejvs.2013.02.014

[10] Azhar A, Basheer M, Abdelgawad MS, Roshdi H, Kamel MF. Prevalence of peripheral arterial disease in diabetic foot ulcer patients and its impact in limb salvage. The International Journal of Lower Extremity Wounds. 2021;**2021**:1-6. DOI: 10.1177/15347346211027063

[11] Kaminski MR, Lambert KA, Raspovic A, McMahon LP, Erbas B, Mount PF, et al. Risk factors for foot ulceration in adults with end-stage renal disease on dialysis: A prospective observational cohort study. BMC Nephrology. 2019;**20**(1):1-11. DOI: 10.1186/s12882-019-1594-5

[12] Sage RA, Pinzur M, Stuck R, Napolitano C. Amputation and Rehabilitation of the Diabetic Foot. Diabetic Foot. Totowa, NJ: Humana Press; 2007. pp. 363-389. DOI: 10.1007/978-1-59745-075-1_18

[13] Huang YY, Lin CW, Yang HM, Hung SY, Chen IW. Survival and associated risk factors in patients with diabetes and amputations caused by infectious foot gangrene. Journal of Foot and Ankle Research. 2018;**11**(1):1-7. DOI: 10.1186/s13047-017-0243-0

[14] Woldemariam GT, Atnafu NT, Radie YT, Wolde GT, Gebreagziabher TT, Gebrehiwot TG, et al. Determinants of diabetic foot ulcer among adult patients with diabetes attending the diabetic clinic in tikur anbessa specialized hospital, Addis ababa, Ethiopia: Unmatched case–control study. Diabetes, Metabolic Syndrome and Obesity. 2020;**13**:3739-3747. DOI: 10.2147/DMSO.S265988

[15] Pemayun TGD, Naibaho RM, Novitasari D, Amin N, Minuljo TT. Risk factors for lower extremity amputation in patients with diabetic foot ulcers: A hospital-based case-control study. Diabetic Foot & Ankle. 2015;**6**:1-12. DOI: 10.3402/dfa.v6.29629

[16] Pitocco D, Spanu T, Di Leo M, Vitiello R, Rizzi A, Tartaglione L, et al. Diabetic foot infections: A comprehensive overview. European Review for Medical and Pharmacological Sciences. 2019;**23**(2):26-37. DOI: 10.26355/EURREV_201904_17471

[17] Everett E, Mathioudakis N. Update on management of diabetic foot ulcers. Annals of the New York Academy of Sciences. 2018;**1411**(1):153-165. DOI: 10.1111/nyas.13569

[18] Alexiadou K, Doupis J. Management of diabetic foot ulcers. Diabetes Therapy. 2012;**3**(1):1-15. DOI: 10.1007/s13300-012-0004-9

[19] Tappia PS, Hiebert B, Sanjanwala R, Komenda P, Sathianathan C, Arneja AS, et al. A novel bathing therapeutic approach for diabetic foot ulcers. Applied Sciences. 2021;**11**(18):1-13. DOI: 10.3390/app11188402

[20] Smith-Strøm H, Iversen MM, Igland J, Østbye T, Graue M, Skeie S, et al. Severity and duration of diabetic foot ulcer (DFU) before seeking care as predictors of healing time: A retrospective cohort study. PLoS One. 2017;**12**(5):1-15. DOI: 10.1371/journal.pone.0177176

[21] Noor S, Zubair M, Ahmad J. Diabetic foot ulcer—A review on pathophysiology, classification and microbial etiology. Diabetes and Metabolic Syndrome: Clinical Research and Reviews. 2015;**9**(3):192-199. DOI: 10.1016/j.dsx.2015.04.007

[22] Abu-Qamar MZ, Kemp V, Whitehead L. Foot ulcers associated with external trauma among people with diabetes: An integrative review of the origin of trauma and outcomes. International Journal of Nursing Studies. 2021;**114**:103822. DOI: 10.1016/j.ijnurstu.2020.103822

[23] Calvet HM, Yoshikawa TT. Infections in diabetes. Infectious Disease Clinics of North America. 2001;**15**(2):407-421. DOI: 10.1016/S0891-5520(05)70153-7

[24] Vincent AM, Russell JW, Low P, Feldman EL. Oxidative stress in the pathogenesis of diabetic neuropathy. Endocrine Reviews. 2004;**25**(4):612-628. DOI: 10.1210/er.2003-0019

[25] Kobayashi M, Zochodne DW. Diabetic neuropathy and the sensory neuron: New aspects of pathogenesis and their treatment implications. Journal of Diabetes Investigation. 2018;**9**(6):1239-1254. DOI: 10.1111/jdi.12833

[26] Ristikj-Stomnaroska D, Risteska-Nejashmikj V, Papazova M. Role of inflammation in the pathogenesis of diabetic peripheral neuropathy. Open Access Macedonian Journal of Medical Sciences. 2019;**7**(14):2267-2270. DOI: 10.3889/oamjms.2019.646

[27] Mizukami H, Osonoi S, Takaku S, Yamagishi SI, Ogasawara S, Sango K, et al. Role of glucosamine in development of diabetic neuropathy independent of the aldose reductase pathway. Brain Communications. 2020;**2**(2):1-18. DOI: 10.1093/braincomms/fcaa168

[28] DiNicolantonio JJ, O'Keefe HJ. Myo-inositol for insulin resistance, metabolic syndrome, polycystic ovary syndrome and gestational diabetes. Open Heart. 2022;**9**(1):1-7. DOI: 10.1136/openhrt-2022-001989

[29] Grover M, Makkar R, Sehgal A, Seth SK, Gupta J, Behl T. Etiological aspects for the occurrence of diabetic neuropathy and the suggested measures. Neurophysiology. 2020;**52**(2):159-168. DOI: 10.1007/s11062-020-09865-2

[30] Grennan D. Diabetic foot ulcers. Journal of the American Medical Association. 2019;**321**:1. DOI: 10.1001/jama.2018.18323

[31] Lechner A, Akdeniz M, Tomova-Simitchieva T, Bobbert T, Moga A, Lachmann N, et al. Comparing skin characteristics and molecular markers of xerotic foot skin between diabetic and non-diabetic subjects: An exploratory study. Journal of Tissue Viability. 2019;**28**(4):200-209. DOI: 10.1016/j.jtv.2019.09.004

[32] Shashikumar C, Alshammari QT. The risk association between foot complications and duration in type 2 diabetes mellitus. International Journal of Diabetes & Metabolic Disorders. 2021;**6**(2):194-197

[33] Theocharidis G, Veves A. Autonomic nerve dysfunction and impaired diabetic wound healing: The role of neuropeptides. Autonomic Neuroscience. 2020;**223**:102610. DOI: 10.1016/j.autneu.2019.102610

[34] Kumar S, Tan Y, Berthiaume F. Neuropeptide substance P enhances skin wound healing in vitro and in vivo under hypoxia. Biomedicine. 2021;**9**(2):1-12. DOI: 10.3390/biomedicines9020222

[35] Alavi A, Sibbald RG, Mayer D, Goodman L, Botros M, Armstrong DG, et al. Diabetic foot ulcers: Part I. pathophysiology and prevention. Journal of the American Academy of Dermatology. 2014;**70**(1):1.e1-1.e18. DOI: 10.1016/j.jaad.2013.06.055

[36] Odriozola A, Ortega L, Martinez L, Odriozola S, Torrens A, Corroleu D, et al. Widespread sensory neuropathy in diabetic patients hospitalized with severe COVID-19 infection. Diabetes Research and Clinical Practice. 2021;**172**:108631. DOI: 10.1016/j.diabres.2020.108631

[37] Yeboah K, Agyekum JA, Owusu Mensah RNA, Affrim PK, Adu-Gyamfi L, Doughan RO, et al. Arterial stiffness is associated with peripheral sensory neuropathy in diabetes patients in Ghana. Journal Diabetes Research. 2018;**2018**: 1-8. DOI: 10.1155/2018/2320737

[38] Venkataraman K, Tai BC, Khoo EYH, Tavintharan S, Chandran K, Hwang SW, et al. Short-term strength and balance training does not improve quality of life but improves functional status in individuals with diabetic peripheral neuropathy: A randomised controlled trial. Diabetologia. 2019;**62**(12):2200-2210. DOI: 10.1007/s00125-019-04979-7

[39] Chatchawan U, Jarasrungsichol K, Yamauchi J. Immediate effects of self-Thai foot massage on skin blood flow, skin temperature, and range of motion of the foot and ankle in type 2 diabetic patients. Journal of Alternative and Complementary Medicine. 2020;**26**(6):491-500. DOI: 10.1089/acm.2019.0328

[40] Khammash MR, Obeidat KA. Prevalence of ischemia in diabetic foot infection. World Journal of Surgery. 2003;**27**(7):797-799. DOI: 10.1007/s00268-003-6889-8

[41] Pemayun TGD, Naibaho RM, Novitasari D, Amin N, Minuljo TT. Risk factors for lower extremity amputation in patients with diabetic foot ulcers: A hospital-based case-control study. Diabetic Foot & Ankle. 2015;**6**:29629. DOI: 10.3402/dfa.v6.29629

[42] Ugwu E, Adeleye O, Gezawa I, Okpe I, Enamino M, Ezeani I. Predictors of lower extremity amputation in patients with diabetic foot ulcer: Findings from MEDFUN, a multi-center observational study. Journal of Foot and Ankle Research. 2019;**12**(1):1-8. DOI: 10.1186/s13047-019-0345-y

[43] Ikem R, Ikem I, Adebayo O, Soyoye D. An assessment of peripheral vascular disease in patients with diabetic foot ulcer. The Foot. 2010;**20**(4):114-117. DOI: 10.1016/j.foot.2010.09.002

[44] Snow DE, Everett J, Mayer G, Cox SB, Miller B, Rumbaugh K, et al. The presence of biofilm structures in atherosclerotic plaques of arteries from legs amputated as a complication of diabetic foot ulcers. Journal of Wound Care. 2016;**25**:S16-S22. DOI: 10.12968/jowc.2016.25.Sup2.S16

[45] Nicholls SJ, Tuzcu EM, Kalidindi S, Wolski K, Moon KW, Sipahi I, et al. Effect of diabetes on progression of coronary atherosclerosis and arterial remodeling. A pooled analysis of 5 intravascular ultrasound trials. Journal of the American College of Cardiology. 2008;**52**(4):255-262. DOI: 10.1016/j.jacc.2008.03.051

[46] Wagenknecht LE, Zaccaro D, Espeland MA, Karter AJ, O'Leary DH, Haffner SM. Diabetes and progression of carotid atherosclerosis: The insulin resistance atherosclerosis study. Arteriosclerosis, Thrombosis, and Vascular Biology. 2003;**23**(6):1035-1041. DOI: 10.1161/01.ATV.0000072273.67342.6D

[47] Tabit CE, Chung WB, Hamburg NM, Vita JA. Endothelial dysfunction in diabetes mellitus: Molecular mechanisms and clinical implications. Reviews in Endocrine & Metabolic Disorders. 2010;**11**(1):61-74. DOI: 10.1007/s11154-010-9134-4

[48] Hamilton SJ, Watts GF. Endothelial dysfunction in diabetes: Pathogenesis, significance, and treatment. The Review of Diabetic Studies. 2013;**10**(2-3):133-156. DOI: 10.1900/RDS.2013.10.133

[49] Vena GA, Cassano N, Di Leo E, Calogiuri GF, Nettis E. Focus on the role of substance P in chronic urticaria. Clinical and Molecular Allergy. 2018;**16**(1):1-6. DOI: 10.1186/s12948-018-0101-z

[50] Sandoval-Talamantes AK, Gómez-González BA, Uriarte-Mayorga DF, Martínez-Guzman MA, Wheber-Hidalgo KA, Alvarado-Navarro A. Neurotransmitters, neuropeptides and their receptors interact with immune response in healthy and psoriatic skin.

Neuropeptides. 2020;**79**:102004. DOI: 10.1016/j.npep.2019.102004

[51] Kumar G, Dey SK, Kundu S. Functional implications of vascular endothelium in regulation of endothelial nitric oxide synthesis to control blood pressure and cardiac functions. Life Sciences. 2020;**259**:118377. DOI: 10.1016/j.lfs.2020.118377

[52] Shimokawa H, Godo S. Nitric oxide and endothelium-dependent hyperpolarization mediated by hydrogen peroxide in health and disease. Basic & Clinical Pharmacology & Toxicology. 2020;**127**(2):92-101. DOI: 10.1111/bcpt.13377

[53] Kosmopoulos M, Drekolias D, Zavras PD, Piperi C, Papavassiliou AG. Impact of advanced glycation end products (AGEs) signaling in coronary artery disease. Biochimica et Biophysica Acta—Molecular Basis of Disease. 2019;**1865**(3):611-619. DOI: 10.1016/j.bbadis.2019.01.006

[54] Robson R, Kundur AR, Singh I. Oxidative stress biomarkers in type 2 diabetes mellitus for assessment of cardiovascular disease risk. Diabetes and Metabolic Syndrome: Clinical Research and Reviews. 2018;**12**(3):455-462. DOI: 10.1016/j.dsx.2017.12.029

[55] Papachristoforou E, Lambadiari V, Maratou E, Makrilakis K. Association of glycemic indices (hyperglycemia, glucose variability, and hypoglycemia) with oxidative stress and diabetic complications. Journal Diabetes Research. 2020;**2020**:7489795. DOI: 10.1155/2020/7489795

[56] Arora D, Kumar M, Dubey SD, Sings U. Immunomodulating effects of rasayana drugs in diabetics—A clinical study. Ancient Science of Life. 2002;**22**(2):42-48

[57] Mishra A, Podder V, Modgil S, Khosla R, Anand A, Nagarathna R, et al. Higher perceived stress and poor glycemic changes in prediabetics and diabetics among Indian population. Journal of Medicine and Life. 2020;**13**(2):132-137. DOI: 10.25122/jml-2019-0055

[58] Hobizal KB, Wukich DK. Diabetic foot infections: Current concept review. Diabetic Foot & Ankle. 2012;**3**:1-8. DOI: 10.3402/dfa.v3i0.18409

[59] Abdulrazak A, Ibrahim Bitar Z, Ayesh Al-Shamali A, Ahmed Mobasher L. Bacteriological study of diabetic foot infections. Journal of Diabetes and its Complications. 2005;**19**(3):138-141. DOI: 10.1016/j.jdiacomp.2004.06.001

[60] Kwon KT, Armstrong DG. Microbiology and antimicrobial therapy for diabetic foot infections. Infection & Chemotherapy. 2018;**50**(1):11-20. DOI: 10.3947/ic.2018.50.1.11

[61] Edmonds M, Manu C, Vas P. The current burden of diabetic foot disease. Journal of Clinical Orthopaedics and Trauma. 2021;**17**:88-93. DOI: 10.1016/j.jcot.2021.01.017

[62] Paschou SA, Stamou M, Vuagnat H, Tentolouris N, Jude E. Pain management of chronic wounds: Diabetic ulcers and beyond. Maturitas. 2018;**117**:17-21. DOI: 10.1016/j.maturitas.2018.08.013

[63] Noor S, Raghav A, Parwez I, Ozair M, Ahmad J. Molecular and culture based assessment of bacterial pathogens in subjects with diabetic foot ulcer. Diabetes and Metabolic Syndrome: Clinical Research and Reviews. 2018;**12**(3):417-421. DOI: 10.1016/j.dsx.2018.03.001

[64] Jiang D, Scharffetter-Kochanek K. Mesenchymal stem cells adaptively respond to environmental cues thereby improving granulation tissue formation and wound healing. Frontiers in Cell and Development Biology. 2020;**8**:1-13. DOI: 10.3389/fcell.2020.00697

[65] Kartika RW, Alwi I, Suyatna FD, Yunir E, Waspadji S, Immanuel S, et al. The use of image processing in the evaluation of diabetic foot ulcer granulation after treatment with advanced-platelet rich fibrin + hyaluronic acid. Systematic Reviews in Pharmacy. 2020;**11**(12):519-526. DOI: 10.31838/srp.2020.12.84

[66] Marshall A, Alam U, Themistocleous A, Calcutt N, Marshall A. Novel and emerging electrophysiological biomarkers of diabetic neuropathy and painful diabetic neuropathy. Clinical Therapeutics. 2021;**43**(9):1441-1456. DOI: 10.1016/j.clinthera.2021.03.020

[67] Ramirez-Acuña JM, Cardenas-Cadena SA, Marquez-Salas PA, Garza-Veloz I, Perez-Favila A, Cid-Baez MA, et al. Diabetic foot ulcers: Current advances in antimicrobial therapies and emerging treatments. Antibiotics. 2019;**8**(4):1-32. DOI: 10.3390/antibiotics8040193

[68] Heravi FS, Zakrzewski M, Vickery K, Armstrong DG, Hu H. Bacterial diversity of diabetic foot ulcers: Current status and future prospectives. Journal of Clinical Medicine. 2019;**8**(11):1935. DOI: 10.3390/jcm8111935

[69] Zubair M. Prevalence and interrelationships of foot ulcer, risk-factors and antibiotic resistance in foot ulcers in diabetic populations: A systematic review and meta-analysis. World Journal of Diabetes. 2020;**11**(3):78-89. DOI: 10.4239/wjd.v11.i3.78

[70] Matta-Gutiérrez G, García-Morales E, García-Álvarez Y, Álvaro-Afonso FJ, Molines-Barroso RJ, Lázaro-Martínez JL. The influence of multidrug-resistant bacteria on clinical outcomes of diabetic foot ulcers: A systematic review. Journal of Clinical Medicine. 2021;**10**(9):1948. DOI: 10.3390/jcm10091948

[71] Malik A, Morya RK, Saha S, Singh PK, Bhadada SK, Rana SV. Oxidative stress and inflammatory markers in type 2 diabetic patients. European Journal of Clinical Investigation. 2020;**50**(6):2-7. DOI: 10.1111/eci.13238

[72] Jin L, Zhang J, Deng Z, Liu J, Han W, Chen G, et al. Mesenchymal stem cells ameliorate myocardial fibrosis in diabetic cardiomyopathy via the secretion of prostaglandin E2. Stem Cell Research & Therapy. 2020;**11**(1):1-13. DOI: 10.1186/s13287-020-01633-7

[73] Koye DN, Magliano DJ, Nelson RG, Pavkov ME. The global epidemiology of diabetes and kidney disease. Advances in Chronic Kidney Disease. 2018;**25**(2):121-132. DOI: 10.1053/j.ackd.2017.10.011

[74] Kovesdy CP. Epidemiology of chronic kidney disease: An update 2022. Kidney International. Supplement (2011). 2022;**12**(1):7-11. DOI: 10.1016/j.kisu.2021.11.003

[75] Alicic RZ, Rooney MT, Tuttle KR. Diabetic kidney disease: Challenges, progress, and possibilities. Clinical Journal of the American Society of Nephrology. 2017;**12**(12):2032-2045. DOI: 10.2215/CJN.11491116

[76] Chammas NK, Hill RLR, Edmonds ME. Increased mortality in diabetic foot ulcer patients:

The significance of ulcer type. Journal Diabetes Research. 2016;**2016**:2879809. DOI: 10.1155/2016/2879809

[77] Manenti L, Tansinda P, Vaglio A. Uraemic pruritus. Drugs. 2009;**69**(3):251-263. DOI: 10.2165/00003495-200969030-00002

[78] Budisavljevic MN, Cheek D, Ploth DW. Calciphylaxis in chronic renal failure. Journal of the American Society of Nephrology. 1996;**7**(7):978-982. DOI: 10.1681/ASN.V77978

[79] Chrysochou C, Power A, Shurrab AE, Husain S, Moser S, Lay J, et al. Low risk for nephrogenic systemic fibrosis in nondialysis patients who have chronic kidney disease and are investigated with gadolinium-enhanced magnetic resonance imaging. Clinical Journal of the American Society of Nephrology. 2010;**5**(3):484-489. DOI: 10.2215/CJN.06580909

[80] Peng T, Zhuo L, Wang Y, Jun M, Li G, Wang L, et al. Systematic review of sodium thiosulfate in treating calciphylaxis in chronic kidney disease patients. Nephrology. 2018;**23**(7):669-675. DOI: 10.1111/nep.13081

[81] Daudén E, Oñate MJ. Calciphylaxis. Dermatologic Clinics. 2008;**26**(4):557-568. DOI: 10.1016/j.det.2008.05.006

[82] Gaisne R, Péré M, Menoyo V, Hourmant M, Larmet-Burgeo D. Calciphylaxis epidemiology, risk factors, treatment and survival among French chronic kidney disease patients: A case-control study. BMC Nephrology. 2020;**21**(1):1-11. DOI: 10.1186/s12882-020-01722-y

[83] Lewis S, Raj D, Guzman NJ. Renal failure: Implications of chronic kidney disease in the management of the diabetic foot. Seminars in Vascular Surgery. 2012;**25**(2):82-88. DOI: 10.1053/j.semvascsurg.2012.04.007

[84] Pliquett RU, Schwock J, Paschke R, Achenbach H. Calciphylaxis in chronic, non-dialysis-dependent renal disease. BMC Nephrology. 2003;**4**:1-5. DOI: 10.1186/1471-2369-4-8

[85] Raskin NH. Neurological aspects of renal failure. In: Aminoff MJ, editor. Neurology and General Medicine. 2nd ed. New York: Churchill Livingstone; 1995. pp. 303-319

[86] Krishnan AV, Kiernan MC. Uremic neuropathy: Clinical features and new pathophysiological insights. Muscle & Nerve. 2007;**35**:273-290. DOI: 10.1002/mus.20713

[87] Kato S, Chmielewski M, Honda H, Pecoits-Filho R, Matsuo S, Yuzawa Y, et al. Aspects of immune dysfunction in end-stage renal disease. Clinical Journal of the American Society of Nephrology. 2008;**3**:1526-1533. DOI: 10.2215/CJN.00950208

[88] Anding K, Gross P, Rost JM, Allgaier D, Jacobs E. The influence of uraemia and haemodialysis on neutrophil phagocytosis and antimicrobial killing. Nephrology, Dialysis, Transplantation. 2003;**18**:2067-2073. DOI: 10.1093/ndt/gfg330

[89] Opatrny K Jr. Clinical importance of biocompatibility and its effect on haemodialysis treatment. Nephrology, Dialysis, Transplantation. 2003;**18**:S41-S44. DOI: 10.1093/ndt/gfg1044

[90] Stenvinkel P, Ketteler M, Johnson RJ, Lindholm B, Pecoits-Filho R, Riella M, et al. IL-10, IL-6, and TNF-alpha: Central factors in the altered cytokine network of uremia—The good, the bad, and the ugly. Kidney International. 2005;**67**:1216-1233. DOI: 10.1111/j.1523-1755.2005.00200.x

[91] Wattanakit K, Folsom AR, Selvin E, Coresh J, Hirsch AT, Weatherley BD. Kidney function and risk of peripheral arterial disease: Results from the Atherosclerosis Risk in Communities (ARIC) Study. Journal of the American Society of Nephrology. 2007;**18**:629-636. DOI: 10.1681/ASN.2005111204

[92] O'Hare AM, Vittinghoff E, Hsia J, Shlipak MG. Renal insufficiency and the risk of lower extremity peripheral arterial disease: Results from the heart and estrogen/progestin replacement study (HERS). Journal of the American Society of Nephrology. 2004;**15**:1046-1051. DOI: 10.1097/01.asn.0000119574.27772.fd

[93] Guerrero-Romeo F, Rodriguez-Moran M. Relationship of microalbuminuria with the diabetic foot ulcers in type II diabetes. Journal of Diabetes and its Complications. 1998;**12**:193-196. DOI: 10.1016/s1056-8727(97)00112-8

[94] Margolis DJ, Hofstad O, Feldman HI. Association between renal failure and foot ulcer or lower-extremity amputation in patients with diabetes. Diabetes Care. 2008;**31**:1331-1336. DOI: 10.2337/dc07-2244

[95] Hill MN, Feldman HI, Hilton SC, Holechek MJ, Ylitalo M, Benedict GW. Risk of foot complications in long-term diabetic patients with and without ESRD: A preliminary study. ANNA Journal. 1996;**23**:381-386

[96] Morbach S, Quante C, Ochs HR, Gaschler F, Pallast JM, Knevels U. Increased risk of lower-extremity amputation among Caucasian diabetic patients on dialysis. Diabetes Care. 2001;**24**:1689-1690. DOI: 10.2337/diacare.24.9.1689

[97] Wolf G, Müller N, Busch M, Eidner G, Kloos C, Hunger-Battefeld W, et al. Diabetic foot syndrome and renal function in type 1 and 2 diabetes mellitus show close association. Nephrology, Dialysis, Transplantation. 2009;**24**:1896-1901. DOI: 10.1093/ndt/gfn724

[98] Eggers PW, Gohdes D, Pugh J. Nontraumatic lower extremity amputations in the Medicare end-stage renal disease population. Kidney International. 1999;**56**:1524-1533. DOI: 10.1046/j.1523-1755.1999.00668.x

[99] Deery HG II, Sangeorzan JA. Saving the diabetic foot with special reference to the patient with chronic renal failure. Infectious Disease Clinics of North America. 2001;**15**:953-981. DOI: 10.1016/s0891-5520(05)70179-3

[100] Griffiths GD, Wieman TJ. The influence of renal function on diabetic foot ulceration. Archives of Surgery. 1990;**125**:1567-1569. DOI: 10.1001/archsurg.1990.01410240045010

[101] Yasuhara H, Naka S, Yanagie H, Nagawa H. Influence of diabetes on persistent nonhealing ischemic foot ulcer in endstage renal disease. World Journal of Surgery. 2002;**26**:1360-1364. DOI: 10.1007/s00268-002-6335-3

[102] Miyajima S, Shirai A, Yamamoto S, Okada N, Matsushita T. Risk factors for major limb amputations in diabetic foot gangrene patients. Diabetes Research and Clinical Practice. 2006;**71**:272-279. DOI: 10.1016/j.diabres.2005.07.005

[103] Stone PA, Back MR, Armstrong PA, Flaherty SK, Keeling WB, Johnson BL, et al. Midfoot amputations expand limb salvage rates for diabetic foot infections. Annals of Vascular Surgery. 2005;**19**:805-811. DOI: 10.1007/s10016-005-7973-3

[104] Pollard J, Hamilton GA, Rush SM, Ford LA. Mortality and morbidity after transmetatarsal amputation:

Retrospective review of 101 cases. The Journal of Foot and Ankle Surgery. 2006;**45**:91-97. DOI: 10.1053/j.jfas.2005.12.011

[105] Young BA, Maynard C, Reiber G, Boyko EJ. Effects of ethnicity and nephropathy on lower-extremity amputation risk among diabetic veterans. Diabetes Care. 2003;**26**:495-501. DOI: 10.2337/diacare.26.2.495

[106] Malik J, Kudlicka J, Lachmanova J, Valerianova A, Rocinova K, Bartkova M, et al. Tissue ischemia worsens during hemodialysis in end-stage renal disease patients. The Journal of Vascular Access. 2017;**18**(1):47-51. DOI: 10.5301/jva.5000630

[107] Pruijm M, Hofmann L, Vogt B, Muller ME, Piskunowicz M, Stuber M, et al. Renal tissue oxygenation in essential hypertension and chronic kidney disease. International Journal of Hypertension. 2013;**2013**:696598. DOI: 10.1155/2013/696598

[108] Singh P, Ricksten SE, Bragadottir G, Redfors B, Nordquist L. Renal oxygenation and haemodynamics in acute kidney injury and chronic kidney disease. Clinical and Experimental Pharmacology & Physiology. 2013;**40**(2):138-147. DOI: 10.1111/1440-1681.12036

[109] Priyadarshi A, Shapiro JI. Erythropoietin resistance in the treatment of the anemia of chronic renal failure. Seminars in Dialysis. 2006;**19**(4):273-278. DOI: 10.1111/j.1525-139X.2006.00172.x

[110] Bosman DR, Osborne CA, Marsden JT, Macdougall IC, Gardner WN, Watkins PJ. Erythropoietin response to hypoxia in patients with diabetic autonomic neuropathy and non-diabetic chronic renal failure. Diabetic Medicine. 2002;**19**(1):65-69. DOI: 10.1046/j.1464-5491.2002.00634.x

[111] Duscher D, Januszyk M, Maan ZN, Whittam AJ, Hu MS, Walmsley GG, et al. Comparison of the hydroxylase inhibitor dimethyloxalylglycine and the iron chelator deferoxamine in diabetic and aged wound healing. Plastic and Reconstructive Surgery. 2017;**139**(3):695e-706e. DOI: 10.1097/PRS.0000000000003072

[112] Moens S, Goveia J, Stapor PC, Cantelmo AR, Carmeliet P. The multifaceted activity of VEGF in angiogenesis—Implications for therapy responses. Cytokine & Growth Factor Reviews. 2014;**25**(4):473-482. DOI: 10.1016/j.cytogfr.2014.07.009

[113] Przybylski M. A review of the current research on the role of bFGF and VEGF in angiogenesis. Journal of Wound Care. 2009, 2009;**18**(12):516-519. DOI: 10.12968/jowc.2009.18.12.45609

[114] Ndip A, Lavery LA, Boulton AJ. Diabetic foot disease in people with advanced nephropathy and those on renal dialysis. Current Diabetes Reports. 2010;**10**(4):283-290. DOI: 10.1007/s11892-010-0128-0

[115] Game FL, Chipchase SY, Hubbard R, Burden RP, Jeffcoate WJ. Temporal association between the incidence of foot ulceration and the start of dialysis in diabetes mellitus. Nephrology, Dialysis, Transplantation. 2006;**21**(11):3207-3210. DOI: 10.1093/ndt/gfl427

[116] Kaminski MR, Raspovic A, McMahon LP, Strippoli GF, Palmer SC, Ruospo M, et al. Risk factors for foot ulceration and lower extremity amputation in adults with end-stage renal disease on dialysis: A systematic review and meta-analysis. Nephrology, Dialysis,

Transplantation. 2015;**30**(10):1747-1766. DOI: 10.1093/ndt/gfv114

[117] Allison GM, Flanagin E. How ESKD complicates the management of diabetic foot ulcers: The vital role of the dialysis team in prevention, early detection, and support of multidisciplinary treatment to reduce lower extremity amputations. Seminars in Dialysis. 2020;**33**(3):245-253. DOI: 10.1111/sdi.12875

[118] Ndip A, Lavery LA, Lafontaine J, Rutter MK, Vardhan A, Vileikyte L, et al. High levels of foot ulceration and amputation risk in a multiracial cohort of diabetic patients on dialysis therapy. Diabetes Care. 2010;**33**:878-880. DOI: 10.2337/dc09-2007

[119] Ndip A, Rutter MK, Vileikyte L, Vardhan A, Asari A, Jameel M, et al. Dialysis treatment is an independent risk factor for foot ulceration in patients with diabetes and stage 4 or 5 chronic kidney disease. Diabetes Care. 2010;**33**(8):1811-1816. DOI: 10.2337/dc10-0255

[120] Volaco A, Chantelau E, Richter B, Luther B. Outcome of critical foot ischaemia in longstanding diabetic patients: A retrospective cohort study in a specialised tertiary care Centre. VASA. 2004;**33**:36-41. DOI: 10.1024/0301-1526.33.1.36

[121] McGrath NM, Curran BA. Recent commencement of dialysis is a risk factor for lower-extremity amputation in a highrisk diabetic population. Diabetes Care. 2000;**23**:432-433. DOI: 10.2337/diacare.23.3.432

[122] Speckman RA, Frankenfield DL, Roman SH, Eggers PW, Bedinger MR, Rocco MV, et al. Diabetes is the strongest risk factor for lower-extremity amputation in new hemodialysis patients. Diabetes Care. 2004;**27**:2198-2203. DOI: 10.2337/diacare.27.9.2198

[123] Morbach S, Quante C, Ochs HR, Gaschler F, Pallast JM, Knevels U. Increased risk of lowerextremity amputation among Caucasian diabetic patients on dialysis. Diabetes Care. 2001;**24**:1689-1690. DOI: 10.2337/diacare.24.9.1689

[124] Lavery LA, Hunt NA, Lafontaine J, Baxter CL, Ndip A, Boulton AJ. Diabetic foot prevention: A neglected opportunity in high risk patients. Diabetes Care. 2010;**33**(7):1460-1462. DOI: 10.2337/dc10-0310

[125] Hambleton IR, Jonnalagadda R, Davis CR, Fraser HS, Chaturvedi N, Hennis AJ. All-cause mortality after diabetes-related amputation in Barbados: A prospective case-control study. Diabetes Care. 2009;**32**:306-307. DOI: 10.2337/dc08-1504

[126] George RK, Verma AK, Agarwal A, Mishra SK. An audit of foot infections in patients with diabetes mellitus following renal transplantation. International Journal of Lower Extremity Wounds. 2004;**3**:157-160. DOI: 10.1177/1534734604267768

[127] Kalker AJ, Pirsch JD, Heisey D, Sollinger HW, Belzer FO, Knechtle SJ, et al. Foot problems in the diabetic transplant recipient. Clinical Transplantation. 1996;**10**:503-510

[128] Nyberg G, Hartso M, Mjornstedt L, Norden G. Type 2 diabetic patients with nephropathy in a Skandinavian kidneytransplant population. Scandinavian Journal of Urology and Nephrology. 1996;**30**:317-322. DOI: 10.3109/00365599609182314

[129] Morrissey PE, Shaffer D, Monaco AP, Conway P, Madras PN. Peripheral vascular disease after kidney-pancreas transplantation in diabetic patients with end-stage renal disease. Archives of Surgery.

1997;**132**:358-361. DOI: 10.1001/archsurg.1997.01430280032004

[130] Sharma A, Vas P, Cohen S, Patel T, Thomas S, Fountoulakis N, et al. Clinical features and burden of new onset diabetic foot ulcers post simultaneous pancreas kidney transplantation and kidney only transplantation. Journal of Diabetes and its Complications. 2019;**33**(9):662-667. DOI: 10.1016/j.jdiacomp.2019.05.017

[131] Nelson EA, Wright-Hughes A, Brown S, Lipsky BA, Backhouse M, Bhogal M, et al. Concordance in diabetic foot ulceration: A cross-sectional study of agreement between wound swabbing and tissue sampling in infected ulcers. Health Technology Assessment. 2016;**20**(82):1-176. DOI: 10.3310/hta20820

[132] Nelson EA, Backhouse MR, Bhogal MS, Wright-Hughes A, Lipsky BA, Nixon J, et al. Concordance in diabetic foot ulcer infection. BMJ Open. 2013;**3**(1):e002370. DOI: 10.1136/bmjopen-2012-002370

[133] Dowd SE, Delton Hanson J, Rees E, Wolcott RD, Zischau AM, Sun Y, et al. Survey of fungi and yeast in polymicrobial infections in chronic wounds. Journal of Wound Care. 2011;**20**(1):40-47. DOI: 10.12968/jowc.2011.20.1.40

[134] Shettigar K, Jain S, Bhat DV, Acharya R, Ramachandra L, Satyamoorthy K, et al. Virulence determinants in clinical Staphylococcus aureus from monomicrobial and polymicrobial infections of diabetic foot ulcers. Journal of Medical Microbiology. 2016;**65**(12):1392-1404. DOI: 10.1099/jmm.0.000370

[135] Buch PJ, Chai Y, Goluch ED. Treating polymicrobial infections in chronic diabetic wounds. Clinical Microbiology Reviews. 2019;**32**(2):e00091-e00018. DOI: 10.1128/CMR.00091-18

[136] Wukich DK, Armstrong DG, Attinger CE, Boulton AJ, Burns PR, Frykberg RG, et al. Inpatient management of diabetic foot disorders: A clinical guide. Diabetes Care. 2013;**36**(9):2862-2871. DOI: 10.2337/dc12-2712

[137] Tan TW, Shih CD, Concha-Moore KC, Diri MM, Hu B, Marrero D, et al. Correction: Disparities in outcomes of patients admitted with diabetic foot infections. PLoS One. 2019;**14**(4):e0215532. DOI: 10.1371/journal.pone.0215532

[138] Abbas M, Uçkay I, Lipsky BA. In diabetic foot infections antibiotics are to treat infection, not to heal wounds. Expert Opinion on Pharmacotherapy. 2015;**16**(6):821-832. DOI: 10.1517/14656566.2015.1021780

[139] Balducci S, Sacchetti M, Haxhi J, Orlando G, D'Errico V, Fallucca S, et al. Physical exercise as therapy for type II diabetes. Diabetes/Metabolism Research and Reviews. 2014;**30**(Suppl 1):13-23. DOI: 10.1002/dmrr.2514

[140] Baker N. Debridement of the diabetic foot: A podiatric perspective. The International Journal of Lower Extremity Wounds. 2002;**1**(2):87-92. DOI: 10.1177/1534734602001002003

[141] Kaile K, Mahadevan J, Leiva K, Khandavilli D, Narayanan S, Muthukrishnan V, et al. Tissue oxygenation measurements to aid scalpel debridement removal in patients with diabetes. Journal of Diabetes Science and Technology. 2022;**16**(2):460-469. DOI: 10.1177/1932296821992050

[142] Gianino E, Miller C, Gilmore J. Smart wound dressings for diabetic chronic wounds. Bioengineering (Basel). 2018;**5**(3):51. DOI: 10.3390/bioengineering5030051

[143] Lai HJ, Kuan CH, Wu HC, Tsai JC, Chen TM, Hsieh DJ, et al. Tailored design of electrospun composite nanofibers with staged release of multiple angiogenic growth factors for chronic wound healing. Acta Biomaterialia. 2014;**10**(10):4156-4166. DOI: 10.1016/j.actbio.2014.05.001

[144] Dwivedi C, Pandey I, Pandey H, Patil S, Mishra SB, Pandey AC, et al. In vivo diabetic wound healing with nanofibrous scaffolds modified with gentamicin and recombinant human epidermal growth factor. Journal of Biomedical Materials Research. Part A. 2018;**106**(3):641-651. DOI: 10.1002/jbm.a.36268

[145] Houlind K. Surgical revascularization and reconstruction procedures in diabetic foot ulceration. Diabetes/Metabolism Research and Reviews. 2020;**36**(Suppl 1):e3256. DOI: 10.1002/dmrr.3256

[146] Wang A, Lv G, Cheng X, Ma X, Wang W, Gui J, et al. Guidelines on multidisciplinary approaches for the prevention and management of diabetic foot disease (2020 edition). Burns & Trauma. 2020;**8**:tkaa017. DOI: 10.1093/burnst/tkaa017

[147] Aragón-Sánchez J, Víquez-Molina G, López-Valverde ME, Rojas-Bonilla JM, Murillo-Vargas C. Surgical diabetic foot infections: Is osteomyelitis associated with a worse prognosis? The International Journal of Lower Extremity Wounds. 2021;**2021**:1534734620986695. DOI: 10.1177/1534734620986695

[148] Lipscombe J, Jassal SV, Bailey S, Bargman JM, Vas S, Oreopoulos DG. Chiropody may prevent amputations in diabetic patients on peritoneal dialysis. Peritoneal Dialysis International. 2003;**23**:255-259

[149] Neil JA, Knuckey CJ, Tanenberg RJ. Prevention of foot ulcers in patients with diabetes and end stage renal disease. Nephrology Nursing Journal. 2003;**30**:39-43

[150] Foster AV, Snowden S, Grenfell A, Watkins PJ, Edmonds ME. Reduction of gangrene and amputations in diabetic renal transplant patients: The role of a special foot clinic. Diabetic Medicine. 1995;**12**:632-635. DOI: 10.1111/j.1464-5491.1995.tb00555.x

[151] Uccioli L, Faglia E, Monticone G, Favales F, Durola L, Aldeghi A, et al. Manufactured shoes in the prevention of diabetic foot ulcers. Diabetes Care. 1995;**18**:1376-1378. DOI: 10.2337/diacare.18.10.1376

Chapter 2

Insight of the Pathophysiology of Diabetic Foot Ulcer

Idris Long

Abstract

The implications of prolonged hyperglycaemia in diabetic individuals include an increased incidence of foot ulcers. Prolonged hyperglycaemia creates a toxic environment in diabetes nerves, particularly at the foot. It also contributes to the hypoxic situation in this region. This disorder causes the nerves, particularly those in the foot, to die and become incapable of responding to sensation stimuli. However, the pathogenesis of diabetic foot ulcers is largely unknown. This chapter attempts to describe the aetiology of foot ulcers through peripheral neuropathy, vascular disease, trauma and infection and explore the evaluation and diagnostic criteria and the current therapy and management of diabetic foot ulcers.

Keywords: hyperglycaemia, diabetic foot ulcer, neuropathy, vascular disease, trauma and infection

1. Introduction

Diabetes patients experience diabetic foot ulcer (DFU) as a result of prolonged hyperglycaemia, and it is the most common reason for hospitalisation. It is also associated with severe morbidity and mortality and, if not recognised and treated promptly, can result in limb amputation [1]. It also had an influence on the financial burden placed on patients, their families, society and the government for the treatment and management of DFU [2]. The risk of a patient with diabetes developing a foot ulcer has been estimated to be 19–34%, and the incidence rates for ulcer recurrence remain high which is 40% within 1 year after healing and 65% within 5 years [3].

Hyperglycaemia stimulates enzymes such as aldose reductase and sorbitol dehydrogenase, resulting in the conversion of intracellular glucose to sorbitol and fructose. The accumulation of these converted glucose products reduces the synthesis of myoinositol in nerve cells that are essential for energy production [4]. The chemical change caused by glucose also resulted in the depletion of nicotinamide adenine dinucleotide phosphate (NADP), which is required for the detoxification of reactive oxygen species (ROS) and the synthesis of the vasodilator, nitric oxide (NO). As a result, there is an increase in oxidative stress on nerve cells, as well as an increase in vasoconstriction on blood vessel, which leads to ischemia, which causes nerve cell damage and death [5]. The common sites for ulceration on foot are dorsal or plantar aspects of the toes, plantar metatarsal heads and heel.

There are numerous events in diabetic progress that can contribute to the development of DFU. The most important events are diabetic peripheral neuropathy (DPN), which affects half of all diabetics, peripheral vascular disease (PVD) and trauma and infection [6].

1.1 Diabetic peripheral neuropathy (DPN)

DPN can be sensory, motor or autonomic. Sensory neuropathy reduces the patient's sensory awareness and manifests clinically as burning, tingling or paraesthesia in the stocking and glove distribution, which worsens after numbness symptoms appear [7]. The peripheral nerve fibres in diabetic patients are affected in a length-dependent manner, with the longest nerves being affected first, resulting in a stocking distribution of sensory loss. Sensory loss involving type A myelin fibres results in loss of proprioception, pressure sensation, vibratory perception and gait impairment. The destruction of type C sensory fibres results in an inability to recognise painful stimuli. As a result of these impaired sensations, the diabetic patient may suffer from repetitive foot trauma, such as blister formation or even metatarsal bone fracture, without realising it. Poor balance due to loss of proprioception, decreased sweating and dry skin that can develop skin cracks and fissures are all consequences of DPN [8].

Motor neuropathy can result in structural changes in the shape of the foot. It is typically presents as wasting of the intrinsic muscles of the foot, resulting in clawing of the toes and changes to the architecture of the mid-foot and subsequently in pressure redistribution over the metatarsal heads. Loss of the Achilles reflex is the earliest sign of these changes. With atrophy of the lumbricals and interosseous muscles, the anatomy of the foot arch changes, with a relative increase in extensor tendon forces producing a "claw" deformity of the toes. A shift to extrinsic muscle/tendon function contributes to depression of the metatarsal heads, hammer-toe contracture of the digits and equine ankle deformity [9].

Whereas autonomic neuropathy can impair the microvascular thermoregulation and anhidrosis process that adds to the motor and sensory disturbance. From this malfunction, the skin becomes dry as it loses the ability to moisturise its surface due to decreased secretory functions of the sebaceous and sweat glands and prone to fissuring, diminishes its effectiveness as a barrier to microorganism invasion, becoming susceptible to dermal infection, that is, cellulitis [10].

1.2 Peripheral vascular disease (PVD)

Microvascular and macrovascular diseases are the two types of diabetic vascular complications. Endothelial cellular dysfunction and smooth muscle abnormalities develop in diabetics as a result of a decrease in endothelium-derived vasodilators, resulting in constriction of blood arteries in the foot [11]. In diabetic patients, glucose levels in cells and tissues rise, stimulating glycolytic and polyol pathways in the peripheral nerve. Furthermore, protein modification with Advanced Glycation End-products (AGEs) and AGE accumulation causes structural (nerve fibre loss or demyelination and thickening of the endothelium's basement membrane in microvessel) and functional damage in small fibre nerves and microvessel. This situation is more vulnerable to diabetic patients' distal lower limb microvessel, which typically affects small arteries below the knee and within the foot, resulting in ischaemia at this site. This microcirculatory complication appears much earlier in the stage of prediabetes and worsens over time [12].

Furthermore, macrovascular disease such as atherosclerosis causes blockage in major arteries due to thickening of blood capillaries and hardening of arteriolar walls, and it's also ended up with ischaemia. In DFU, determining the degree of ischaemia is critical. The pedal pulses (dorsalis pedis and posterior tibial arteries) must be carefully palpated. The dorsalis pedis artery is absent or significantly reduced in size in approximately 12% of the population, so a pulse may not be palpable. A cool foot with no palpable pedal pulses should be investigated further with non-invasive arterial Doppler ultrasonography of the lower limb. Beside these, other risk factors can also contribute into PVD such as age, smoking, hypertension, hyperlipidaemia, inflammatory markers and renal dysfunction [13].

1.3 Trauma and infection

Trauma might also contribute to the development of ulceration in DFU. Ill-fitting shoes are the most prevalent source of trauma, and also injuries go missed due to a lack of sensation [14]. Motor neuropathy causes structural changes in the structure of the foot; as a result, many regular shoes are inappropriate for diabetic patients. Walking-related repetitive stress, along with diminished sensation and proprioception, predisposes to skin damage by producing atrophy and displacement of protective plantar fat pads, leading to ulceration and infection with inadequate skin protection or inappropriate footwear [15].

Neglecting skin protection, such as forgetting to apply moisturising lotions or failing to recognise cutaneous stress (redness, blister formation), can lead to ulceration

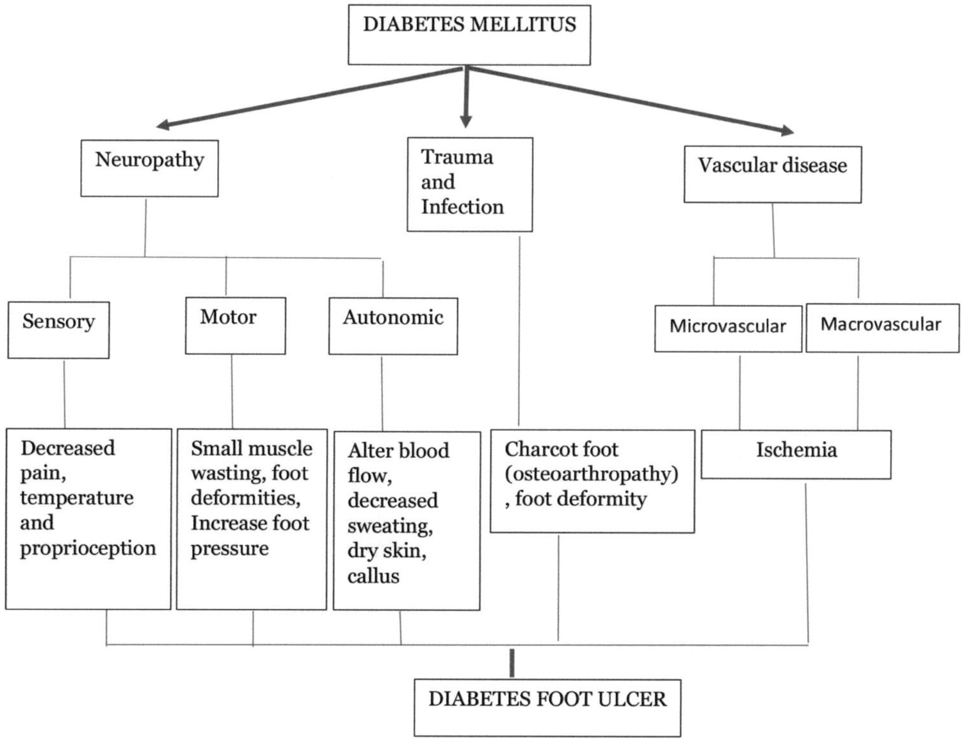

Figure 1.
Common pathway to diabetic foot ulcer.

and the development of an invasive soft-tissue infection. If not treated quickly, tissue degradation will persist, especially if the patient continues to walk. The risk of ulceration increases significantly in the presence of peripheral neuropathy, foot deformity or previous digit amputation (by 32 times) [1].

Trauma in the foot could also lead into infection that penetrates the deep fascia, allowing infection to spread into the mid-foot muscles, joints and tendon sheaths. In diabetics, infection is responsible for 50% of all major (above- or below-knee) lower-extremity amputations. Polymicrobial infections (staphylococci, streptococci, enterococci, Escherichia coli and other Gram-negative bacteria) are widespread, as is the presence of antibiotic-resistant bacterial strains, particularly methicillin-resistant Staphylococcus aureus, which occurs in 30–40% of cases. When a diabetic foot infection contains resistant bacterial strains, which is commonly the result of repeated or protracted antibiotic use, the risk of amputation rises [16]. The common pathway to DFU is illustrated in **Figure 1**.

2. Evaluation and diagnosis of DFU

Diabetic patients need to regularly check their foot from any sign of ulcer and infection. A typical foot examination encompasses four aspects which are dermatologic, vascular, neurologic and musculoskeletal.

2.1 Dermatologic

The dermatologist will look for any thickness or discolouration of the toenails, as well as hyperkeratosis on the toes or balls of the feet. The state of the patient's skin reveals information regarding the health of the patient's feet. Toenails that are excessively swollen, opaque, disintegrating, yellow in colour and malodorous are most likely fungal, indicating sensory, autonomic or both neuropathies. Peripheral neuropathy dulls the sensation and allows patients to bear more sustained pressure on a small region of skin without experiencing pain. Shear pressures induce the skin to react to aberrant stimuli, causing keratinisation to rise. Autonomic neuropathy makes it difficult to maintain normal skin moisture balance and control. The skin becomes either too dry and scaly or too wet, promoting dermatophyte infections and skin maceration inside the webspaces [9, 16, 17].

2.2 Vascular

Palpation of the dorsalis pedis and posterior tibial is part of the vascular examination. Because the dorsalis pedis artery is missing or diminished in size in the majority of diabetes individuals, a palpable pulse cannot be felt. The capillary refill time to each digit is also essential in determining blood flow to the toes and the microvasculature's state. Peripheral oedema may be indicative of autonomic neuropathy caused by venous blood insufficiency in the lower extremities. The lower legs have dark discolouration up to the mid-tibia [18].

2.3 Neurologic

The neurologic evaluation involves testing the patellar and Achilles deep tendon reflexes. The loss of the Achilles reflex is a sign of severe peripheral neuropathy.

Sensitivity is assessed for vibratory loss using a 128 Hz tuning fork, while sensation to light touch is determine using microfilament, pin prick and temperature (tuning fork placed in warm or ice water then applied to dorsum of foot and positional sense in the toes). Neuropathy is characterised by decreased proprioception and a loss of light touch. Balance issues will be revealed by gait analysis. Walking from heel to toe might be challenging with peripheral neuropathy. A patient's larger base of gait may suggest lack of proprioception, and balance may be considerably reduced with the eyes closed. The Romberg test (loss of balance with feet together and eyes closed) is also used when evaluating neuropathy [19].

2.4 Musculoskeletal

The musculoskeletal assessment involves looking for common foot abnormalities such bunions (hallux valgus), constricted toes and Tailor's bunions (lateral exostosis fifth metatarsal head). With the patient upright, clinicians should look for any noticeable asymmetry changes in arch height. Common symptoms of a patient's foot "looking odd" or changing in appearance and becoming red, hot and swollen without any history of trauma to the region should prompt a radiograph and referral to a podiatrist for treatment. Unexplained swelling in the feet is a sign of active Charcot alterations, especially if just one foot is affected. Diabetic foot infection, osteomyelitis and cellulitis, acute inflammatory arthropathy, gout, acute thrombosis and trauma are all causes of a Charcot deformity [20].

2.5 Imaging

In an acute presentation of a DFU, plain radiography is the most frequent first-line radiographic study to check for underlying osteomyelitis. It is cheap and widely available. If feasible, weighty viewpoints should be taken. Radiographs can identify osteomyelitis, osteolysis, fractures, dislocations, medial arterial calcification, soft tissue gas and foreign substances, as well as structural foot abnormalities and the presence of arthritis [20]. CT scans may be used to evaluate suspected bone and joint disease that is not visible on conventional radiography. CT provides excellent anatomic information and resolution of bone, including osseous fragmentation and joint subluxation. Subluxation of the transverse tarsal or tarsometatarsal joints can be seen prior to being visualised on radiographs [21]. Because of its enhanced resolution and ability to visualise the extent of any infectious process, MRI is usually preferred over CT for the investigation of osteomyelitis. MRI is frequently used in evaluating both soft tissue and bone pathology. This scan may be used to help diagnose osteomyelitis, deep abscesses, septic joints and tendon rupture. MRI is particularly sensitive for bone infection and may also be utilised for surgical planning [22].

3. Current therapy and management of DFU

The strategy for the management of patients with a DFU is multidisciplinary approach to address the multifactorial processes involved in DFU. It includes all relevant specialties team such as nursing, orthopaedics, plastic surgery, vascular surgery, nutrition and endocrinology. This approach can decrease the risks DFU and amputation by 50–85%, lowering the cost medication and leading to a better quality of life for patients with DFU.

3.1 Treatments for diabetic peripheral neuropathy (DPN)

Pharmacological treatment is used to control the painful sensation of DPN which manifested as numbness, burning, stabbing or excruciating or intractable pain. The U.S. Food and Drug Administration (FDA) has approved three drugs for the pain associated with DPN, namely, pregabalin, tapentadol and duloxetine. Besides that, analgesics such as tramadol, acetaminophen and opioids such as oxycodone also have been prescribed for pain associated with DPN. However, these drugs produced many sides effect such as constipation and nausea and had high tendency to be misused. Antidepressants such as amitriptyline, nortriptyline and venlafaxine have shown and efficacy in DPN management, but the doses in clinical trial are not reproducible in clinical practice [22].

Antioxidants such as Alpha-lipoic acid (ALA) have been shown to be a possible treatment agent for DPN by delaying or reversing nerve damage [23]. Treatments based on mesenchymal stem cell (MSC) generated from adipose tissue might potentially be regarded as possible DPN treatments. These medicines increase the production of pro-angiogenic, neuroprotective and anti-inflammatory substances, which improves the clinical presentation of the illness [24]. Biological treatment with lower doses of IL-6 also can help increase blood flow, reduce chronic inflammation, repair peripheral nerve fibre and restore DPN peripheral nerve function [25].

3.2 Treatments for peripheral vascular disease (PVD).

In diabetic patients, a decrease in blood flow in both the microvascular (capillaries) and macrovascular (arteries and veins) systems, as well as a decrease in angiogenesis, raises the risk of ischemia. Tissue ischemia manifesting as dependent rubor with rest discomfort, ulceration or gangrene necessitates rapid examination for correctable artery occlusive disease in order to enhance perfusion and save limbs. In general, all patients with foot lesions and vascular testing revealing an ankle pressure of 100 mm Hg or toe pressure of 55 mm Hg should have arterial imaging investigations performed to identify occlusive lesions amenable to revascularisation such as open bypass or endovascular treatment [14]. In cases of common femoral artery occlusion, bypass is more successful and provides extended patency. Whereas, endovascular treatment similar to angioplasty in which a tiny balloon is inserted into a constricted portion of an artery and inflated to open the artery to enhance blood flow in the lower extremities [26]. Atherectomy is another method that uses a spinning cutting blade to remove atheroma. Diabetic patients must get multidisciplinary care, including medication for hypertension, hypercholesterolemia and bleeding, in order for these procedures to be effective [27].

3.3 Relief of foot pressure

The persistent and recurrent traumatism of the foot, as well as the use of inappropriate footwear, contributes to the development of a DFU. Both lower extremities should be inspected for skin trauma (redness, induration, oedema), ulceration, foot/toe deformity and popliteal and ankle (posterior tibial, dorsalis pedis) pulses palpated. The education on precise foot care and suitable footwear must be stressed in the diabetic patient. Diabetic patients should be taught to self-examine their skin and feet on a regular basis, as well as be educated on skin care and footwear management [28].

3.4 Infection treatment

Antibiotic treatment for DFU will be administered based on the pathogen that is most likely causing the infection and the severity of the illness. It can be tweaked based on the findings of the microbiological culture and the treatment's effectiveness. The duration of antibiotic treatment is determined by the severity of the illness; for example, a moderate infection might be treated for 1–2 weeks, a severe infection for 2–4 weeks and osteomyelitis for longer [29]. Dicloxacillin, cephalexin, clindamycin and amoxicillin/clavulanate are recommended antibiotics for mild-moderate cases; vancomycin + ampicillin/sulbactam, moxifloxacin, cefoxitin or cefotetan for moderate cases, and vancomycin + piperacillin/tazobactam, imipenem/cilastatin, meropenem or doripenem for severe cases [29, 30, 31].

3.5 Tissue engineering approaches

Tissue engineering is a regenerative medicine discipline that combines growth factors, cells and scaffolds to restore, preserve or improve damaged tissues or whole organs [32]. Growth factors are proteins that promote and activate cell proliferation by stimulating angiogenesis and the transcription of certain genes. Growth factors such as epidermal growth factor (EGF), platelet-derived growth factor (PDGF), fibroblast growth factor (FGF), transforming growth factor beta (TGF) and vascular endothelial growth factor (VEGF) are examples of growth factors. All of these growth factors have been shown to be beneficial in DFU tissue healing [33]. Cells obtained from bone marrow and umbilical cord blood such as mesenchymal stem cells (MSCs), fibroblasts and keratinocytes have also been employed for tissue repair in DFU [33, 34, 35]. Furthermore, biomaterials derived from natural resources such as collagen, hyaluronic acid, fibrin, chitosan and alginate, as well as synthetic materials such as poly (acrylic acid) (PAA), polyglycolic acid (PGA), PCL-poly (ethylene glycol) (PEG), gelatin methacrylate (GelMA) have been used as hydrogels, bandages, foam and films in DFU treatment. These biomaterials have been recommended for used in DFU treatment because of their ease of degradation, good biocompatibility and resistance to the scaffolding material [36].

4. Conclusions

DFU frequently results in complications such as infection, osteomyelitis, abscesses and amputations of the lower extremities. It also has a significant influence on patients' physical, psychological, social and economic elements, as well as their overall quality of life. The pathophysiology of DFU, on the other hand, is still unknown. It is critical to understand the pathophysiology of DFU in order to properly treat and manage the condition. Several causes, including diabetic peripheral neuropathy (DPN), which affects 50% of all diabetics, peripheral vascular disease (PVD) and trauma and infection, have been identified as critical events for DFU to develop. Many biological therapeutic remedies have been produced as a result of technical advances to help in the healing process of DFU. Tissue engineering is a revolutionary therapy for DFU that has the potential to lead to new treatments in the future.

Acknowledgements

This study was supported by the Fundamental Research Grant Scheme (FRGS) Ministry of Higher Education Malaysia (FRGS/1/2020/SKK0/USM/03/5).

Declaration of conflicting interests

The author(s) declared no potential conflicts of interest concerning the research, authorship and/or publication of this article.

Author details

Idris Long
School of Health Sciences, Universiti Sains Malaysia, Kubang Kerian, Malaysia

*Address all correspondence to: idriskk@usm.my

References

[1] Boulton AJM. The diabetic foot. Med (United Kingdom). 2019;**47**(2):100-5

[2] Raghav A, Khan ZA, Labala RK, Ahmad J, Noor S, Mishra BK. Financial burden of diabetic foot ulcers to world: A progressive topic to discuss always. Therapeutic Advances in Endocrinology and Metabolism. 2018;**9**(1):29-31

[3] Armstrong DG, Boulton AJM, Bus SA. Diabetic foot ulcers and their recurrence. The New England Journal of Medicine. 2017;**376**(24):2367-2375

[4] Brownlee M. The pathobiology of diabetic complications: A unifying mechanism. Diabetes. 2005;**54**(6):1615-1625

[5] Clayton W, Elasy TA. Patofizjologia, klasyfikacja i leczenie owrzodzeń stóp u chorych na cukrzycę. Diabetol Prakt 2009. 2009;**10**(5):211-212

[6] Reardon R, Simring D, Kim B, Mortensen J, Williams D, Leslie A. The diabetic foot ulcer. AJGP-05-2020-Focus-Reardon-Diabetic-Foot-Ulcer-WEB. 2020;**49**(5):250-255

[7] Forlee M. What is the diabetic foot?: Main article. CME : Your SA Journal of CPD. 2011;**29**(1):4-8

[8] Balasubramanian G, Vas P, Chockalingam N, Naemi R. A synoptic overview of neurovascular interactions in the foot. Front Endocrinol (Lausanne). 2020;**11**(May):1-11

[9] Alavi A, Sibbald RG, Mayer D, Goodman L, Botros M, Armstrong DG, et al. Diabetic foot ulcers: Part I. Pathophysiology and prevention. Journal of the American Academy of Dermatology. 2014;**70**(1):1.e1-1.e18

[10] Boulton AJM. Diabetic neuropathy and foot complications. In: Zochodne DW, Malik RA, editors. Handbook of Clinical Neurology. 1st ed. Vol. 126. Diabetes and the Nervous System. Amsterdam: Elsevier BV; 2014. pp. 97-107

[11] Li XY. Peripheral arterial disease. Chinese Medical Journal. 2014;**127**(4):68-70

[12] Janka HU, Standl E, Mehnert H. Peripheral vascular disease in diabetes mellitus and its relation to cardiovascular risk factors: Screening with the Doppler ultrasonic technique. Diabetes Care. 1980;**3**(2):207-213

[13] Giannopoulos S, Armstrong EJ. Diabetes mellitus: An important risk factor for peripheral vascular disease. Expert Review of Cardiovascular Therapy. 2020;**18**(3):131-137

[14] Balducci S, Sacchetti M, Haxhi J, Orlando G, D'Errico V, Fallucca S, et al. Physical exercise as therapy for type II diabetes. Diabetes/Metabolism Research and Reviews. 2014;**32**(30):13-23

[15] Kim PJ, Attinger CE, Evans KK, Steinberg JS. Role of the podiatrist in diabetic limb salvage. Journal of Vascular Surgery. 2012;**56**(4):1168-1172

[16] Bandyk DF. The diabetic foot: Pathophysiology, evaluation, and treatment. Seminars in Vascular Surgery. 2018;**31**(2-4):43-48

[17] Bowling FL, Rashid ST, Boulton AJM. Preventing and treating foot complications associated with diabetes mellitus. Nature Reviews. Endocrinology. 2015;**11**(10):606-616

[18] Boulton AJM. Peripheral neuropathy and the diabetic foot. The Foot. 1992;**2**(2):67-72

[19] Handsaker JC, Brown SJ, Bowling FL, Marple-Horvat DE, Boulton AJM, Reeves ND. People with diabetic peripheral neuropathy display a decreased stepping accuracy during walking: Potential implications for risk of tripping. Diabetic Medicine. 2016;**33**(5):644-649

[20] Peterson N, Widnall J, Evans P, Jackson G, Platt S. Diagnostic imaging of diabetic foot disorders. Foot & Ankle International. 2017;**38**(1):86-95

[21] Ergen FB, Sanverdi SE, Oznur A. Charcot foot in diabetes and an update on imaging. Diabet Foot Ankle. 2013;**4**

[22] Nóbrega MBDM, Aras R, Netto EM, Couto RD, Marinho AMDN, da Silva JL, et al. Risk factors for charcot foot. The Archives of Endocrinology and Metabolism. 2015;**59**(3):226-230

[23] Vallianou N, Evangelopoulos A, Koutalas P. Alpha-lipoic acid and diabetic neuropathy. The Review of Diabetic Studies. 2009;**6**(4):230-236

[24] Oses C, Olivares B, Ezquer M, Acosta C, Bosch P, Donoso M, et al. Preconditioning of adipose tissue-derived mesenchymal stem cells with deferoxamine increases the production of pro-angiogenic, neuroprotective and anti-inflammatory factors: Potential application in the treatment of diabetic neuropathy. PLoS One. 2017;**12**(5):1-22

[25] Cox AA, Sagot Y, Hedou G, Grek C, Wilkes T, Vinik AI, et al. Low-dose pulsatile interleukin-6 as a treatment option for diabetic peripheral neuropathy. Front Endocrinol (Lausanne). (MAY):2017;**8**(89). DOI: 10.3389/fendo.2017.00089

[26] Uccioli L, Meloni M, Izzo V, Giurato L, Merolla S, Gandini R. Vascular health and risk management dovepress critical limb ischemia: Current challenges and future prospects. Vascular Health and Risk Management. 2018;**14**:63-74

[27] Gatti C, Cecchini S, Fabbietti P, Romagnoli F, Ricci S. Endovascular treatment of diabetic peripheral arterial disease in older and oldest old patients: A retrospective study. Aging Clinical and Experimental Research. 2018;**30**(2):205-207

[28] Fleischli JG, Lavery LA, Vela SA, Ashry H, Lavery DC. Stickel Bronze Award. Comparison of strategies for reducing pressure at the site of neuropathic ulcers. Journal of the American Podiatric Medical Association. 1997;**87**(10):466-472

[29] Grigoropoulou P, Eleftheriadou I, Jude EB, Tentolouris N. Diabetic foot infections: An update in diagnosis and management. Current Diabetes Reports. 2017;**17**(1):3

[30] Bowling FL, Boulton AJM. Neuropathy D. Diabetic foot Diabetic Foot. 2022:1-7

[31] Singh S, Gupta B. Choices and challenges of antibiotics therapy in diabetic foot infection. Indian Journal of Endocrinology and Metabolism. 2017;**21**(5):647-648

[32] Katari R, Peloso A, Orlando G. Tissue engineering and regenerative medicine: Semantic considerations for an evolving paradigm. Frontiers in Bioengineering and Biotechnology. 2015;**2**(January):1-6

[33] João De Masi ECD, Campos ACL, João De Masi FD, Ratti MAS, Ike IS, João De Masi RD. A influência de fatores de crescimento na cicatrização de feridas cutâneas de ratas. Brazilian Journal of Otorhinolaryngology. 2016;**82**(5):512-521

[34] Cao Y, Gang X, Sun C, Wang G. Mesenchymal stem cells improve healing of diabetic foot ulcer. Journal Diabetes Research. 2017;**2017**:10. Article ID: 9328347. DOI: org/10.1155/2017/9328347

[35] Werner S, Krieg T, Smola H. Keratinocyte-fibroblast interactions in wound healing. The Journal of Investigative Dermatology. 2007;**127**(5).998-1008

[36] Tottoli EM, Dorati R, Genta I, Chiesa E, Pisani S, Conti B. Skin wound healing process and new emerging technologies for skin wound care and regeneration. Pharmaceutics. 2020;**12**(8):1-30

Section 2

Treatment

Chapter 3

Macrophages as a Target for Treating Diabetic Foot Ulcers

Lingyan Zhu, Yu Xiao, Yao Xiao, Yinan Jiang, Maharana Prathap Adama and George K. Gittes

Abstract

In all stages of wound healing, macrophages play a pivotal role by coordinating the repair steps in a timely and accurate fashion. The successful completion of wound healing requires proper spatiotemporal presence and function of macrophages. Diabetes significantly alters the proliferation, polarization and functionality of macrophages, leading to a suboptimal but prolonged pro-inflammatory M1-like phenotype in wound macrophages and a failure of their late transition to a reparative M2-like phenotype. This defect in macrophage phenotype and the proper transition results in delayed or even failure of wound healing. Specifically in the diabetic foot ulcer (DFUs), this macrophage dysfunction results in chronic infection and potentially amputation. The abnormal macrophage phenotype in diabetes is not fully understood but is believed to mainly result from epigenetic changes in macrophages and altered interactions between macrophages and other cell types, such as fibroblasts, endothelial cells, neutrophils and T-cells. Recent research on DFUs has focused on developing strategies to improve diabetic wound repair through modulation of macrophage polarization. Treatment of DFUs will greatly benefit from a multi-modal therapy that includes controlling high blood glucose, topical support, prevention of secondary infection, resolution of sustained inflammation and application of cellular therapies targeting macrophages.

Keywords: diabetic foot ulcer, diabetic wound healing, macrophage polarization, epigenetics, inflammation

1. Introduction

Diabetes is a metabolic disease that affects over 300 million people worldwide [1]. Diabetes is characterized by high blood glucose levels due to inadequate amounts of insulin produced and secreted by pancreatic beta cells, plus the loss of sensitivity to insulin in peripheral tissues [2]. There are two major types of diabetes, type 1 diabetes (T1D) and type 2 diabetes (T2D) [3]. T1D constitutes about 5% of all diabetes and is known as a T-cell mediated autoimmune invasion and destruction of insulin-producing beta cells in the pancreas, characterized by a significantly reduced beta cell mass and a significantly reduced secretion of insulin [4]. T2D accounts for about 90% of diabetes, and results from the failure of beta cells to compensate for the insensitivity of cells in responsive to insulin, which is called insulin resistance [5].

IntechOpen

Diabetic patients can develop severe complications due to impairment in cell proliferation, differentiation, migration, immune responses, angiogenesis, etc., under a sustained hyperglycemic status [6]. Non-healing wounds, or diabetic foot ulcers (DFUs), are one of the most severe diabetic complications, and represent the leading cause of amputations, with an associated greater than 50% 5-year mortality [7]. Correspondingly, the treatment of DFUs comprises the highest annual US medical expenditure for any diagnosis [8]. Therefore, great effort has been made to understand the pathological processes during diabetic wound healing and to create novel therapies.

During the study of the mechanisms underlying diabetes-related impaired wound healing, accumulating evidence suggests that macrophages play a pivotal role in orchestrating proper wound healing [9]. In the early stages of normal wound healing, macrophages polarize to an M1-like phenotype, whereby they remove pathogens, dead cells and debris, and promote inflammation through secreting pro-inflammatory cytokines [10]. Later in the repair process, macrophages transition to more of an M2-like phenotype to resolve the inflammation and secrete trophic factors that promote the proliferation, differentiation and migration of fibroblasts, keratinocytes, mesenchymal cells and vascular endothelial cells, leading to tissue regeneration, neovascularization and wound repair [10]. These wound macrophages originate from different sources and interact with several other cell types through which they develop diverse functions to properly and efficiently assist with the repair process [11]. It is noteworthy that in diabetes there are alterations in the baseline function of macrophages, as well as the corresponding phenotypic changes in macrophages during the wound healing process [10]. Early in wound healing macrophages are responsible for the initiation and progression of inflammation and removal of pathogens, dead cells and debris. However, at later stages, macrophages instead contribute to the resolution of inflammation, reorganization of extracellular matrices (ECM), re-epithelialization, angiogenesis, cell and tissue regeneration and tissue remodeling through secreting a number of factors at late stages [12]. In a normal healthy situation, macrophages initially polarize to a pro-inflammatory M1 subtype to assist in the early stages of wound healing but then re-polarize to an alternative anti-inflammatory M2 subtype to assist in the later stages of wound healing [13]. Interestingly, diabetes leads to impairment of the M1-to-M2 transition in the later stages of wound healing, resulting in sustained inflammation and compromised cell proliferation, differentiation and migration, abnormal immune responses and inadequate angiogenesis [14]. Therefore, different strategies have been generated to target macrophages in order to reverse this pathologic inflammation during diabetic wound healing through modulating macrophage polarization [15]. In this book chapter, we discuss the role of macrophages in normal wound healing and their impairments during diabetic wound healing. We also discuss the present approaches to enhancing the repair of DFUs through targeting macrophages.

2. Macrophages and their role in inflammation

Neutrophils, macrophages and other cells involved in the innate immune system constitute a first line of defense against microorganisms and are critical for the control and resolution of common infections [16]. However, not all infectious organisms can be recognized by macrophages, for which lymphocytes of the adaptive immune system are present to create a more versatile defense system [17]. The innate and adaptive immune systems cooperate through many interactions among different cell types. For example, cells of the innate immune system such as macrophages, dendritic cells and natural killer (NK) cells orchestrate the initiation and the subsequent progression of lymphocyte-mediated adaptive immune responses, and then receive feedback signaling from lymphocytes to adapt their phenotypes and functions for the direct involvement in the removal of pathogens targeted by adaptive immune responses [18]. Moreover, the innate immune response by macrophages is the critical response to control infections before the adaptive immune response takes effect a few days after the infection [19]. Furthermore, macrophages also contribute to directing the adaptive immune response through antigen presentation and production and secretion of cytokines and chemokines [20].

Classical macrophages display a pro-inflammatory phenotype, which has been designated as "M1" macrophages, while another subtype of macrophages that are alternatively differentiated and exhibit anti-inflammatory properties or contribute to resolution of inflammation, tissue regeneration and remodeling, have been designated as "M2" macrophages [21]. The overall M1 or M2 characteristics in a given macrophage is called its "polarization" [22]. When a macrophage changes its expression pattern to fit a more M1 or M2 phenotype, it is called a polarized macrophage [22]. Macrophage polarization can either occur in undifferentiated macrophages (naïve macrophages) or occur in polarized macrophages, which is then called "re-polarization" [22]. It is now known that polarization of macrophages into the precise definition of "M1" or "M2" macrophages rarely occurs. Instead, macrophage typically polarize into a wide spectrum of phenotypes that exhibit distinct gene and protein expression patterns [23]. This broad range of differentiation pattern allows macrophages to perform diverse tasks throughout the body [23]. M1 macrophages are characterized by high levels of proinflammatory markers such as reactive oxygen species (ROS), inducible nitric oxide synthase (iNOS), nitric oxide (NO), CD11c, tumor necrosis factor (TNF)α, interleukin (IL)-6, IL-1β and major histocompatibility complex (MHC)-II [24]. In contrast, M2 macrophages express markers associated with healing and inhibition of inflammation such as high levels of arginase 1, CD163, CD206, CD301, IL-10, resistin-like molecule alpha1 (Fizz1) and chitinase-like protein 3 (Ym1) [25]. Microenvironmental autocrine and paracrine signals, together with epigenetic changes, seem to influence macrophage activation and polarization [26].

3. The role of macrophages in normal wound healing

Wound healing is a very complex process encompassing 4 specific phases: hemostasis, inflammation, proliferation and remodeling. A successful wound closure requires the process to be well orchestrated by multiple cell types including keratinocytes, fibroblasts, endothelial cells, mesenchymal cells and inflammatory cells (macrophages, lymphocytes, neutrophils, NK cells, etc.) in a dynamic interactive way [10]. These 4 phases occur in a coordinated, linear and partially overlapping manner, in which one earlier phase is required for the completion of later phases [11]. The hemostasis phase is initiated immediately after injury, which involves vasoconstriction, platelet aggregation and activation of the clotting cascade resulting in clot formation and degranulation of platelets to convert soluble fibrinogen to insoluble fibrin and to release factors like P-selectin to recruit neutrophils to initiate the inflammatory phase [27, 28]. Next, the recruited neutrophils (peaking at 2 days after injury) release ROS, antimicrobial peptides and neutrophil extracellular traps in addition to chemokines to attract monocytes/macrophages [27]. Meanwhile, tissue-resident macrophages and other antigen-presenting cells like dendritic cells are activated and release factors [11]. The monocytes/macrophages from either the tissue or the circulation thus become the cell type dominating the inflammatory phase and are the central regulators of this inflammatory phase [29]. Here, the macrophages interact with many cell types, activate a number of signaling pathways, and release many soluble mediators, such as growth factors, chemokines, cytokines and metabolites that signal to other cell types. Thus, the macrophages orchestrate the complex tasks and biological activities to enhance wound healing [30]. At this phase of wound healing, which typically lasts 3 days, macrophages are mainly pro-inflammatory, or M1-like, and produce cytokines such as IL-1β, IL-6, IL-12 and TNFα [10]. However, as early as day 1 after initiation of wound healing, anti-inflammatory or M2-like macrophages start to appear and their numbers increase little by little until they become dominant by about 4 days after wounding when the proliferative phase starts [14]. During the proliferative phase, M2-like macrophages (peaking at 7 days after wound) produce and secrete factors to activate fibroblasts and keratinocytes to proliferate, differentiate and migrate to the wound and deposit collagen and other ECM proteins, though keratinocytes start to proliferate immediately after wound due to loss of contact inhibition [13]. Moreover, M2-like macrophages also promote angiogenesis through interactions with vascular endothelial cells [13]. A requirement for macrophages in the activation and functions of fibroblasts at this phase was proven by a study applying macrophage-depletion [31]. Interestingly, a very recent report showed a myeloid origin of about 10% of wound fibroblasts in a mouse skin wounding model, further supporting the important role and plasticity of macrophages during wound healing [32]. The final remodeling phase is the longest phase of wound healing, during which type I collagen gradually replaces type III collagen to increase tensile strength [33].

Macrophages are key regulators for the overall wound repair process [34]. The wound monocytes/macrophages have different origins. Before injury occurs, skin monocytes/macrophages consist of the tissue-resident macrophages as predominantly Langerhans cells in the epidermal layer, and also as dermal macrophages in the dermis [35]. Wounds without macrophages have less cell proliferation, inadequate differentiation, compromised migration, delayed re-epithelialization, impaired angiogenesis and reduced collagen deposition [27]. Moreover, reduced secretion of vascular endothelial growth factor (VEGF)-A and transforming growth factor (TGF)β1 renders the wounds less conducive to angiogenesis and cell proliferation, which are critical for a proper completion of wound repair [36]. The plasticity of macrophages allows them to be first polarized to a pro-inflammatory M1-like phenotype, and then transition or repolarize to an anti-inflammatory M2-like phenotype [29]. Indeed, M1 macrophages are primarily responsible for destruction of pathogens and production and release of inflammatory cytokines in the wound. Meanwhile, M2 macrophages are associated with the late repair and regeneration phases of wound healing, and they are critical for proper angiogenesis, regeneration and remodeling of ECM, cell growth and replacement, production of anti-inflammatory and trophic cytokines and resolution of the inflammation [37]. Actually, as stated above, macrophages are not all polarized uniformly throughout wound healing [23]. At any given time point they may be in a wide spectrum of phenotypes, and only the predominant phenotype presented as the overall macrophage phenotype at any given time in the repair process (**Figure 1**) [10, 23, 29, 38].

Dermal wound healing is a very complex process encompassing 4 specific phases: hemostasis, inflammation, proliferation and remodeling. These 4 phases occur in a coordinated, linear and partially overlapping manner, in which one earlier phase is

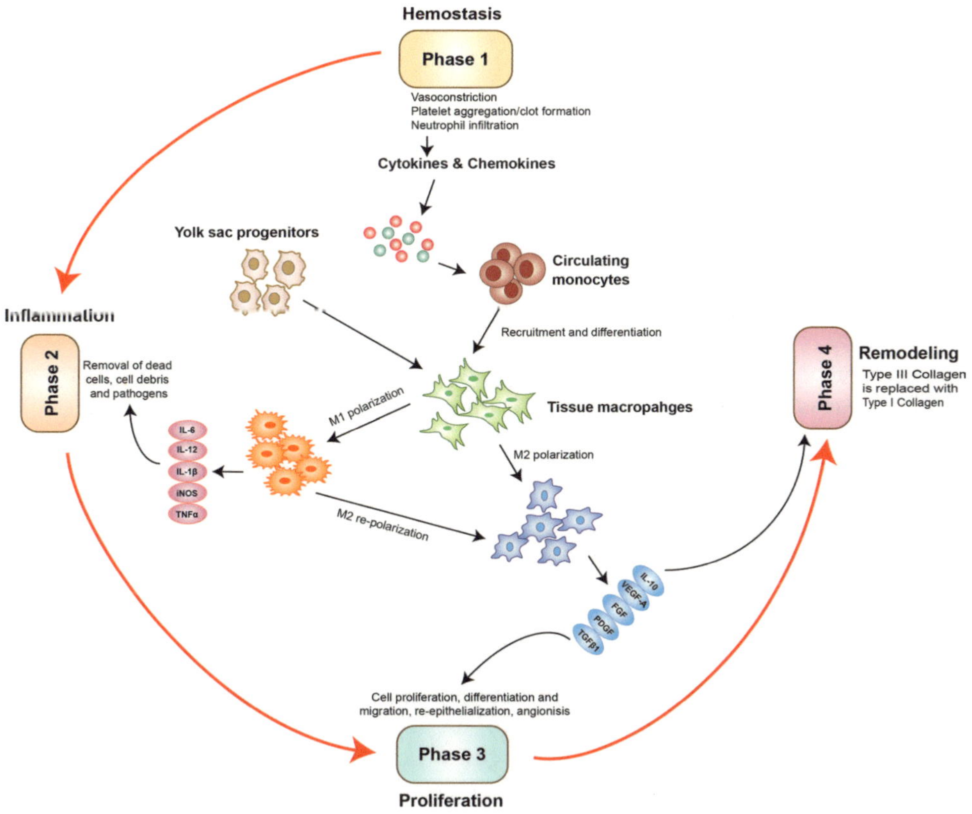

Figure 1.
Role of macrophages in wound healing.

required for the completion of later phases. The hemostasis phase is initiated immediately after injury, and involves vasoconstriction, platelet aggregation and activation of the clotting cascade, resulting in clot formation and degranulation of platelets to convert soluble fibrinogen into insoluble fibrin and to release factors like P-selectin to recruit neutrophils to initiate the inflammatory phase. Next, the recruited neutrophils (peaking at 2 days after injury) release chemokines to attract monocytes/macrophages. Meanwhile, tissue-resident macrophages and other antigen-presenting cells like dendritic cells are activated and release factors. The monocytes/macrophages from either the local tissue or the circulation thus dominate this phase of wound healing, which typically lasts 3 days. At this time, macrophages are mainly pro-inflammatory or M1-like, and produce cytokines such as IL-1β, IL-6, IL-12 and TNFα. However, as early as day 1 after the initiation of wound healing, anti-inflammatory or M2-like macrophages start to appear and their numbers increase little by little until they become dominant by about 4 days after wounding, the point when the proliferative phase starts. In the proliferative phase, M2-like macrophages (peaking at 7 days after wounding) produce and secrete factors to activate fibroblasts and keratinocytes to proliferate, differentiate and migrate to the wound and deposit of collagen and other ECM proteins. Moreover, M2-like macrophages also regulate angiogenesis through interactions with vascular endothelial cells. The final remodeling phase is the longest phase of wound healing, during which type III collagen is gradually replaced with type I collagen to increase tensile strength.

4. Alterations in macrophage polarization in diabetic wounds

Innate immune cells including macrophages have been shown to exhibit a pro-inflammatory phenotype with production and secretion of inflammatory cytokines, factors and chemokines. In diabetic wounds these processes are pathologically exaggerated as a possible contributor to the poorly healing DFU [39]. High susceptibility of diabetic patients to bacterial infections and impaired wound repair is well known [11]. The molecular mechanisms underlying this weakness are not fully understood but have been extensively studied in the past. Now it is believed that disorders in glucose metabolism and related alteration in metabolic pathways may be the reason for this susceptibility [40–42]. Interestingly, for unclear reasons the number of Langerhans and dermal macrophages significantly increases in uninjured diabetic skin [43]. Moreover, the effects of diabetes on macrophages and the related wound healing process are profound, and likely stem from changes in many aspects of the diabetic environment [13, 15, 44–48]. Macrophages that are generated in a high glucose culture system exhibit a reduction in their phagocytic potential and are less capable of clearing an infection [49, 50]. Furthermore, macrophages derived from diabetic mice and human patients appear to have increased responsiveness to inflammatory stimulants and secrete more proinflammatory cytokines than normal, which seems to prevent their later transition into the more reparative M2-like phenotype [51–55]. Indeed, at the initiation of wound healing, the phagocytotic capacity of diabetic M1 macrophages is reduced due to suboptimal differentiation, which happens before the impaired transition of M1 macrophages to M2-like macrophages later on [49, 50]. The failure of their transition or repolarization in the later stages of wound healing prevents regeneration and the repair process, resulting in a delay or even failure to heal [12].

The mechanisms underlying these alterations in the diabetic macrophage phenotype have been extensively studied. Hyperglycemia affects macrophage polarization in vitro and in vivo [46, 56–62]. For example, it has been shown that diabetic mice or human patients have an increased ratio of chemokine (C-C motif) receptor (CCR7) to CD48 3 days after wound formation [46]. CCR7 is an M1 macrophage marker whereas CD48 is an M2 macrophage marker [24]. Moreover, M1 macrophages in diabetes express less matrix metalloproteinases 1 (MMP1) and more pro-inflammatory cytokines like TNFα, resulting in an impairment in keratinocyte migration and subsequent delay of wound repair [46]. Furthermore, a hyperglycemic environment has been shown to lead to an increase in many pro-inflammatory cytokines, including TNFα, IL-1β, IL-12 and IL-6 [63], rendering these M1 macrophages more metabolically active and pro-inflammatory, but less phagocytic [63, 64]. This specific alteration in the phenotype of M1 macrophages under hyperglycemic conditions further increases the sensitivity of macrophages to cytokine stimulation and starts a vicious cycle that maintains M1 macrophage polarization and leads to a prolonged inflammation during the wound healing process [64, 65].

The role of interleukins in macrophage differentiation and polarization has been recently studied [66–73]. Some interleukins have been targeted in a therapeutic modality, exhibiting a significant impact on treatment outcomes. For example, depletion of a pro-inflammatory cytokine, IL-23, causes a significant increase in M2 macrophage polarization through loss of IL-17, which leads to improvements in diabetic wound healing [74]. Similar results have been obtained using IL-17-knockout mice or using antisera against IL-17 [74]. IL-1β is highly expressed in activated M1 macrophages in a hyperglycemic environment [63, 64]. Interestingly, experiments have shown that IL-1β expression is regulated by a protein complex called NOD-, LRR- and pyrin domain-containing protein 3 (NLRP3), which is an inflammasome [75] that controls the dimerization and activation of caspase-1, leading to the subsequent transformation of the IL-1β precursor (pro-IL-1β) into its activated form IL-1β to be secreted [76]. Knockdown of NLRP3 with siRNA-mediated gene silencing reduced the production and secretion of IL-1β, which is beneficial to diabetic wound healing [77].

Recent research has also shed light on epigenetic alterations in macrophages in a hyperglycemic environment. These epigenetic changes can induce enhanced expression of proinflammatory cytokines to promote and sustain M1 macrophage polarization [78]. Now it is believed that epigenetic modifications are the main cause of the alterations in macrophage phenotype in diabetes [79]. The epigenetic modifications include histone modifications, DNA modifications and other post-transcriptional controls like microRNAs [10]. Moreover, regulation of macrophage polarization requires interactions with other cell types such as adipocytes, keratinocytes, fibroblasts and other immune cells (Neutrophils, T-cells, dendritic cells, etc.) that secrete factors to modulate macrophage polarization [14]. In the setting of diabetes, these cell-cell interactions are altered, leading to a suboptimal polarization of macrophages [46, 80–82].

A specific role for histone modification in the control of macrophage polarization has been recently highlighted. In eukaryotes, DNA and histones gather together to generate units called nucleosomes [83]. When histones are tightly wrapped with DNA, the access to transcriptional machinery is blocked to prevent transcription [84]. However, when DNA-histone machinery is disassembled, transcriptional binding is allowed. An N-terminal "tail" with lysine (K) residues on histones can be modified by some enzymes through catalyzing methylation and acetylation [84]. Histone methylation and demethylation are controlled by histone methyltransferases (HMTs) and histone demethylases (HDMs), respectively, which regulate macrophage differentiation and polarization [84] and are responsible for the M1 to M2 repolarization during wound healing [85]. For example, mixed-lineage leukemia 1 (MLL1) is a methyltransferase that catalyzes H3K4me3 deposition to affect macrophage polarization and the induction of expression of proinflammatory genes in macrophages [86]. Mechanistically, MLL1 is found to regulate changes in macrophages partially via Toll-like receptor 4 (TLR4) in both diabetic humans and diabetic mice [87, 88]. On the other hand, Suppressor of variegation, Enhancer of Zeste, Trithorax and myeloid-Nervy-DEAF-1 domain-containing protein 3 (SMYD3), which is another H3K4me3 methyltransferase, has been shown to regulate M2-like polarization of macrophages [89]. Besides HMTs, HDMs also play a critical role in macrophage polarization during wound healing. For example, Jumonji domain-containing protein 3 (JMJD3) is a H3K27 demethylase that regulates a context-dependent polarization of macrophages towards either a proinflammatory M1-like or an anti-inflammatory M2-like macrophage phenotype [90–95]. JMJD3-mediated release of H3K27me3 is compromised in diabetic wound macrophages, resulting in enhanced and sustained expression of genes associated with inflammation [96, 97]. However, lipopolysaccharides (LPS) and IL-4 have been shown to induce JMJD3 for directing M2-like macrophage polarization [96]. Together, a lot of data have demonstrated the importance of histone methylation and demethylation by HMTs and HDMs in controlling macrophage polarization during wound repair [98, 99]. Transcriptional repression is often regulated by DNA methylation, which is catalyzed by DNA methyltransferases (DNMTs) to transfer a methyl group to the cytosine ring of DNA at clusters of CpG islands [100]. The potential binding of transcription factors to a promoter region is significantly altered via methylation of CpG islands on the promoter [101]. For example, DNMT1 has been shown to induce M1-like polarization of macrophages [102]. Moreover, genetic depletion of DNMT1 or chemical suppression of DNMT1 by 5-aza-2′-deoxycytidine promotes M2-like macrophage polarization [103] and improves wound healing in diabetic mice [104]. Macrophage polarization during wound healing has also been shown to be affected by histone acetylation and deacetylation. Transcriptional activation is enhanced by acetylation of the lysine residue on the histone tail, for which an acetyl group is transferred from acetyl CoA to the lysine residue catalyzed by histone acetyltransferases (HATs) [105]. In diabetes, it has been shown that histone deacetylase 6 (HDAC6) alters the phenotype of macrophages through IL-1β but not IL-10 [106].

Post-transcriptional control is also an important regulator of macrophage polarization in diabetes. For example, microRNAs have been shown to be important regulators of gene expression during macrophage polarization [9]. MicroRNAs (miRNAs) are non-coding small RNAs about 20 base pairs in length. miRNAs control protein levels of an expressed gene through Watson-Crick pairing to the 3′-untranslated region (3′-UTR) of the mRNA of a specific gene, resulting in altered protein translation [107]. It has been reported that M2 macrophages express high levels of miRNA-146, while M1 macrophages express low levels of miRNA-146 [108, 109], and the levels of miR-146 appear to alter macrophage polarization and their production and secretion of proinflammatory and anti-inflammatory cytokines [108, 109]. It has also been shown that miR-155 can induce an M1-like macrophage polarization through suppressing antagonists of proinflammatory cytokines [110]. Moreover, miR-33 was shown to favor M2 macrophage polarization through suppressing NLRP3 [111], a key inducer of IL-1β and inflammation [76, 77]. Similarly, long noncoding RNAs (lncRNAs) have an emerging role in regulating macrophage polarization [112–116]. Besides miRNAs, long non-coding RNAs also play essential roles in macrophage phenotypic determination and control of inflammation [117]. The role of lncRNA GASS in macrophage polarization and associated wound healing has been reported recently [113].

5. Strategies to improve diabetic wound healing through manipulating macrophages

DFUs will likely require multimodal therapies for optimal treatment. Novel therapeutics are being generated, including specific targeting of macrophages. Since the initial trigger of all the macrophage defects in diabetes appears to be sustained high blood glucose, correction of the primary problem, the hyperglycemia, would appear to be the first approach to treat problems related to diabetic wound healing [7]. However, only half of diabetics can reach the recommend standard hemoglobin A1c (HbA1c) level of <7.0% (issued by the American Diabetes Association (ADA)) [118]. Thus, it is important to search for novel therapies beyond control of blood glucose [7].

Insulin administration is a regular and effective therapy for those unresponsive to diet changes or non-insulin medications. Insulin has been found to reduce the number of M1 macrophages. Moreover, insulin has been shown to induce M1 to M2 macrophage polarization through peroxisome proliferator-activated receptor-gamma (PPAR-γ) and phosphatidylinositol-3 kinase (PI3K)/Protein kinase B (Akt)/Ras-related C3 botulinum toxin substrate 1 (Rac-1) signaling pathways [47]. Interestingly, the PPAR-γ pathway that reduces proinflammatory cytokine expression and enhances M2 macrophage polarization in normal wound healing is impaired in diabetes and could be partially recovered by insulin [119]. Metformin is a commonly used medication for diabetes. Metformin treatment has been shown to increase M2 macrophages and decrease M1 macrophages [120–125], likely through NLRP3 inflammasome suppression, which was discussed above [123]. Melatonin is a medication not for diabetes. However, it was found to affect macrophage polarization in diabetic wound, likely through effects on insulin [47, 126].

Treatment of chronic wounds benefits largely from localized therapies, which have the advantage of avoiding systemic effects and allowing for local and direct treatment [127]. A hydrocolloid dressing to provide moisture to the wound has been shown to improve M1-to-M2 macrophage transition to favor wound healing, especially in diabetes [128]. In another study, use of a modified dressing in diabetic mice led to an earlier appearance of M2 macrophages at the wound [129]. Thus, certain dressings to induce an M2 macrophage polarization appear to be an attractive strategy for treating chronic diabetic wounds. These dressings help the wounds heal through moisture provision, prevention of infection, induction of anti-inflammatory effects and generation of trophic factors. Along with these dressing benefits, Collagenase Santyl Ointment (CSO), with an important component called Clostridial collagenase, has been shown to increase local expression of IL-10 and arginase 1 that are both critical for M2-like macrophage polarization and functionality [130]. Another modified collagen gel has also been shown to increase IL-10 expression and macrophage migration, resulting in a substantial increase in M2 macrophages in the wound at different time points [128]. In addition, increases in IL-10 expression have also been detected after use of docosahexaenoic acid to treat diabetic wounds, with the therapeutic outcome correlated to the degree of M2 macrophage polarization [45, 131, 132].

Multipotent stem cells (MSCs) have been used in the treatment of DFUs, taking advantage of the capacity of MSCs to differentiate into different cell types such as endothelial cells, fibroblasts and smooth muscle cells that are critical for wound healing. These newly formed cells can produce and secrete trophic factors like VEGF-A, fibroblast growth factor (FGF) and platelet-derived growth factor (PDGF) [133–135]. Recently, we have reported that human MSCs express high levels of miR-205-5p, which inhibits protein translation of VEGF-A through 3'-UTR interactions [136]. Expressing antisense of miR-205-5p (as-miR-205-5p) in human MSCs significantly improved the therapeutic effects of human MSCs on diabetic wound healing in rodent models [136]. Next, we reported that MALAT1 is a lncRNA acting as a competing endogenous RNA (ceRNA) for miR-205-5p and is absent in human MSCs [137]. Expression of MALAT1 significantly attenuated the high expression of miR-205-5p in human MSCs, resulting in upregulation of VEGF-A production and improved therapeutic effects of human MSCs on diabetic wound repair [137]. Of note, these improvement in treating diabetic wounds through increasing VEGF-A levels in human MSCs was shown to be associated with increased vascularization of the wounds [136, 137]. Macrophages express high levels of VEGF receptor 1 (VEGFR1), which is one of the major receptors on macrophages to respond to chemoattractants. Thus, it is possible that the therapeutic effects of increased VEGF-A levels in human MSCs may be due, at least partially, to alterations in macrophage proliferation, differentiation and polarization [21]. Further studies of the exact alterations in macrophages caused by VEGF-A are needed. We have recently shown that another VEGF family member, placental growth factor (PlGF), is capable of altering macrophage migratory capacity and polarization [138]. Moreover, we and others have recently shown that PlGF is decreased in DFUs [139, 140]. PlGF injection significantly improved angiogenesis and diabetic wound healing, with both positive effects being abolished by macrophage-specific depletion of VEGF1R to block the effects of PlGF on macrophages [139]. Together, these approaches showed promise as strategies for treating diabetic wound through targeting macrophages.

6. Conclusions

The treatment of diabetic wounds will benefit from a multi-modal approach including control of hyperglycemia, topical treatment, prevention of secondary infection and inflammation and cellular therapy targeting macrophages.

Acknowledgements

We appreciate the help from Dr. Xiangwei Xiao from Children's Hospital of Pittsburgh, USA, for his critical advice and proofreading during the preparation of this book chapter. This work was supported by grants from the National Natural Science Foundation of China (NO: 81860153 and 81500589), Key Project of Natural Science Foundation of Jiangxi Province (NO: 20202ACBL216007), Key project of Jiangxi Provincial Department of Education (NO: GJJ180021), all awarded to Dr. Lingyan Zhu.

Conflict of interest

The authors declare no conflict of interest.

Author details

Lingyan Zhu[1*], Yu Xiao[1,2], Yao Xiao[1,2], Yinan Jiang[2], Maharana Prathap Adama[2] and George K. Gittes[2]

1 Department of Endocrinology, the First Affiliated Hospital of NanChang University, Nanchang, China

2 Department of Surgery, Children's Hospital of Pittsburgh, University of Pittsburgh School of Medicine, Pittsburgh, PA, USA

*Address all correspondence to: zly982387@126.com

References

[1] Bluestone JA, Herold K, Eisenbarth G. Genetics, pathogenesis and clinical interventions in type 1 diabetes. Nature. 2010;**464**(7293):1293-1300

[2] Charles MA, Leslie RD. Diabetes: Concepts of beta-cell organ dysfunction and failure would lead to earlier diagnoses and prevention. Diabetes. 2021;**70**(11):2444-2456

[3] Pipeleers D, Chintinne M, Denys B, Martens G, Keymeulen B, Gorus F. Restoring a functional beta-cell mass in diabetes. Diabetes, Obesity & Metabolism. 2008;**10**(Suppl 4):54-62

[4] Rodriguez-Calvo T, Chen YC, Verchere CB, Haataja L, Arvan P, Leete P, et al. Altered beta-cell prohormone processing and secretion in type 1 diabetes. Diabetes. 2021;**70**(5):1038-1050

[5] Mezza T, Cinti F, Cefalo CMA, Pontecorvi A, Kulkarni RN, Giaccari A. Beta-cell fate in human insulin resistance and type 2 diabetes: A perspective on islet plasticity. Diabetes. 2019;**68**(6):1121-1129

[6] Ali MK, Pearson-Stuttard J, Selvin E, Gregg EW. Interpreting global trends in type 2 diabetes complications and mortality. Diabetologia. 2022;**65**(1):3-13

[7] American DA. 11. Microvascular complications and foot care: Standards of Medical Care in Diabetes-2021. Diabetes Care. 2021;**44**(Suppl 1):S151-S167

[8] Manickum P, Mashamba-Thompson T, Naidoo R, Ramklass S, Madiba T. Knowledge and practice of diabetic foot care - A scoping review. Diabetes and Metabolic Syndrome: Clinical Research and Reviews. 2021;**15**(3):783-793

[9] Rahmannia M, Amini A, Chien S, Bayat M. Impact of photobiomodulation on macrophages and their polarization during diabetic wound healing: A systematic review. Lasers in Medical Science. 2022 [Online ahead of print]

[10] Wolf SJ, Melvin WJ, Gallagher K. Macrophage-mediated inflammation in diabetic wound repair. Seminars in Cell & Developmental Biology. 2021;**119**:111-118

[11] Barman PK, Koh TJ. Macrophage dysregulation and impaired skin wound healing in diabetes. Frontiers in Cell and Development Biology. 2020;**8**:528

[12] Aitcheson SM, Frentiu FD, Hurn SE, Edwards K, Murray RZ. Skin wound healing: Normal macrophage function and macrophage dysfunction in diabetic wounds. Molecules. Aug 13, 2021;**26**(16):4917

[13] Boniakowski AE, Kimball AS, Jacobs BN, Kunkel SL, Gallagher KA. Macrophage-mediated inflammation in normal and diabetic wound healing. Journal of Immunology. 2017;**199**(1):17-24

[14] Louiselle AE, Niemiec SM, Zgheib C, Liechty KW. Macrophage polarization and diabetic wound healing. Translational Research. 2021;**236**:109-116

[15] Ganesh GV, Ramkumar KM. Macrophage mediation in normal and diabetic wound healing responses. Inflammation Research. 2020;**69**(4): 347-363

[16] Hatano S, Watanabe H. Regulation of macrophage and dendritic cell function by chondroitin Sulfate in innate to

antigen-specific adaptive immunity. Frontiers in Immunology. 2020;**11**:232

[17] Bancroft GJ, Kelly JP, Kaye PM, McDonald V, Cross CE. Pathways of macrophage activation and innate immunity. Immunology Letters. 1994;**43**(1-2):67-70

[18] Hirayama D, Iida T, Nakase H. The phagocytic function of macrophage-enforcing innate immunity and tissue homeostasis. International Journal of Molecular Sciences. Dec 29, 2017;**19**(1):92

[19] Bowdish DM, Loffredo MS, Mukhopadhyay S, Mantovani A, Gordon S. Macrophage receptors implicated in the "adaptive" form of innate immunity. Microbes and Infection. 2007;**9**(14-15):1680-1687

[20] Calandra T, Roger T. Macrophage migration inhibitory factor: A regulator of innate immunity. Nature Reviews. Immunology. 2003;**3**(10):791-800

[21] Sun Y, Li J, Xie X, Gu F, Sui Z, Zhang K, et al. Macrophage-osteoclast associations: Origin, polarization, and subgroups. Frontiers in Immunology. 2021;**12**:778078

[22] Taylor PR, Martinez-Pomares L, Stacey M, Lin HH, Brown GD, Gordon S. Macrophage receptors and immune recognition. Annual Review of Immunology. 2005;**23**:901-944

[23] Nahrendorf M, Swirski FK. Abandoning M1/M2 for a network model of macrophage function. Circulation Research. 2016;**119**(3):414-417

[24] Yunna C, Mengru H, Lei W, Weidong C. Macrophage M1/M2 polarization. European Journal of Pharmacology. 2020;**877**:173090

[25] Lawrence T, Natoli G. Transcriptional regulation of macrophage polarization: Enabling diversity with identity. Nature Reviews. Immunology. 2011;**11**(11):750-761

[26] Ginhoux F, Schultze JL, Murray PJ, Ochando J, Biswas SK. New insights into the multidimensional concept of macrophage ontogeny, activation and function. Nature Immunology. 2016;**17**(1):34-40

[27] Mirza R, DiPietro LA, Koh TJ. Selective and specific macrophage ablation is detrimental to wound healing in mice. The American Journal of Pathology. 2009;**175**(6):2454-2462

[28] Clark RA. Fibrin is a many splendored thing. The Journal of Investigative Dermatology. 2003;**121(5)**:**xxi-xxii**

[29] Minutti CM, Knipper JA, Allen JE, Zaiss DM. Tissue-specific contribution of macrophages to wound healing. Seminars in Cell & Developmental Biology. 2017;**61**:3-11

[30] Hesketh M, Sahin KB, West ZE, Murray RZ. Macrophage phenotypes regulate scar formation and chronic wound healing. International Journal of Molecular Sciences. Jul 17, 2017;**18**(7):1545

[31] Leibovich SJ, Ross R. The role of the macrophage in wound repair. A study with hydrocortisone and antimacrophage serum. The American Journal of Pathology. 1975;**78**(1):71-100

[32] Guerrero-Juarez CF, Dedhia PH, Jin S, Ruiz-Vega R, Ma D, Liu Y, et al. Single-cell analysis reveals fibroblast heterogeneity and myeloid-derived adipocyte progenitors in murine skin wounds. Nature Communications. 2019;**10**(1):650

[33] Eming SA, Wynn TA, Martin P. Inflammation and metabolism in tissue

repair and regeneration. Science. 2017;**356**(6342):1026-1030

[34] Boniakowski AM, denDekker AD, Davis FM, Joshi A, Kimball AS, Schaller M, et al. SIRT3 regulates macrophage-mediated inflammation in diabetic wound repair. The Journal of Investigative Dermatology. 2019;**139**(12):2528-2537 e2522

[35] Ridiandries A, Tan JTM, Bursill CA. The role of chemokines in wound healing. International Journal of Molecular Sciences. Oct 18, 2018;**19**(10):3217

[36] Lucas T, Waisman A, Ranjan R, Roes J, Krieg T, Muller W, et al. Differential roles of macrophages in diverse phases of skin repair. Journal of Immunology. 2010;**184**(7):3964-3977

[37] Liu W, Wang M, Cheng W, Niu W, Chen M, Luo M, et al. Bioactive antiinflammatory antibacterial hemostatic citrate-based dressing with macrophage polarization regulation for accelerating wound healing and hair follicle neogenesis. Bioactive Materials. 2021;**6**(3):721-728

[38] Daley JM, Brancato SK, Thomay AA, Reichner JS, Albina JE. The phenotype of murine wound macrophages. Journal of Leukocyte Biology. 2010;**87**(1):59-67

[39] Kraakman MJ, Murphy AJ, Jandeleit-Dahm K, Kammoun HL. Macrophage polarization in obesity and type 2 diabetes: Weighing down our understanding of macrophage function? Frontiers in Immunology. 2014;**5**:470

[40] Drareni K, Gautier JF, Venteclef N, Alzaid F. Transcriptional control of macrophage polarisation in type 2 diabetes. Seminars in Immunopathology. 2019;**41**(4):515-529

[41] Appari M, Channon KM, McNeill E. Metabolic regulation of adipose tissue macrophage function in obesity and diabetes. Antioxidants & Redox Signaling. 2018;**29**(3):297-312

[42] Ahmed M, de Winther MPJ, Van den Bossche J. Epigenetic mechanisms of macrophage activation in type 2 diabetes. Immunobiology. 2017;**222**(10):937-943

[43] Stojadinovic O, Yin N, Lehmann J, Pastar I, Kirsner RS, Tomic-Canic M. Increased number of Langerhans cells in the epidermis of diabetic foot ulcers correlates with healing outcome. Immunologic Research. 2013;**57**(1-3):222-228

[44] Seraphim PM, Leal EC, Moura J, Goncalves P, Goncalves JP, Carvalho E. Lack of lymphocytes impairs macrophage polarization and angiogenesis in diabetic wound healing. Life Sciences. 2020;**254**:117813

[45] Jia YC, Qiu S, Xu J, Kang QL, Chai YM. Docosahexaenoic acid improves diabetic wound healing in a rat model by restoring impaired plasticity of macrophage progenitor cells. Plastic and Reconstructive Surgery. 2020;**145**(5):942e-950e

[46] Huang SM, Wu CS, Chiu MH, Wu CH, Chang YT, Chen GS, et al. High glucose environment induces M1 macrophage polarization that impairs keratinocyte migration via TNF-alpha: An important mechanism to delay the diabetic wound healing. Journal of Dermatological Science. 2019;**96**(3):159-167

[47] Yu T, Gao M, Yang P, Liu D, Wang D, Song F, et al. Insulin promotes macrophage phenotype transition through PI3K/Akt and PPAR-gamma signaling during diabetic wound healing. Journal of Cellular Physiology. 2019;**234**(4):4217-4231

[48] Kimball AS, Joshi AD, Boniakowski AE, Schaller M, Chung J, Allen R, et al. Notch regulates macrophage-mediated inflammation in diabetic wound healing. Frontiers in Immunology. 2017;**8**:635

[49] Liu BF, Miyata S, Kojima H, Uriuhara A, Kusunoki H, Suzuki K, et al. Low phagocytic activity of resident peritoneal macrophages in diabetic mice: Relevance to the formation of advanced glycation end products. Diabetes. 1999;**48**(10):2074-2082

[50] Rungratanawanich W, Qu Y, Wang X, Essa MM, Song BJ. Advanced glycation end products (AGEs) and other adducts in aging-related diseases and alcohol-mediated tissue injury. Experimental & Molecular Medicine. 2021;**53**(2):168-188

[51] Bannon P, Wood S, Restivo T, Campbell L, Hardman MJ, Mace KA. Diabetes induces stable intrinsic changes to myeloid cells that contribute to chronic inflammation during wound healing in mice. Disease Models & Mechanisms. 2013;**6**(6):1434-1447

[52] Miao M, Niu Y, Xie T, Yuan B, Qing C, Lu S. Diabetes-impaired wound healing and altered macrophage activation: A possible pathophysiologic correlation. Wound Repair and Regeneration. 2012;**20**(2):203-213

[53] Khanna S, Biswas S, Shang Y, Collard E, Azad A, Kauh C, et al. Macrophage dysfunction impairs resolution of inflammation in the wounds of diabetic mice. PLoS One. 2010;**5**(3):e9539

[54] Mirza RE, Fang MM, Ennis WJ, Koh TJ. Blocking interleukin-1beta induces a healing-associated wound macrophage phenotype and improves healing in type 2 diabetes. Diabetes. 2013;**62**(7):2579-2587

[55] Mirza R, Koh TJ. Dysregulation of monocyte/macrophage phenotype in wounds of diabetic mice. Cytokine. 2011;**56**(2):256-264

[56] Gao J, Cheng Y, Hao H, Yin Y, Xue J, Zhang Q, et al. Decitabine assists umbilical cord-derived mesenchymal stem cells in improving glucose homeostasis by modulating macrophage polarization in type 2 diabetic mice. Stem Cell Research & Therapy. 2019;**10**(1):259

[57] Zhao Q, Chu Z, Zhu L, Yang T, Wang P, Liu F, et al. 2-deoxy-d-glucose treatment decreases anti-inflammatory M2 macrophage polarization in mice with tumor and allergic airway inflammation. Frontiers in Immunology. 2017;**8**:637

[58] Izquierdo E, Cuevas VD, Fernandez-Arroyo S, Riera-Borrull M, Orta-Zavalza E, Joven J, et al. Reshaping of human macrophage polarization through modulation of glucose catabolic pathways. Journal of Immunology. 2015;**195**(5):2442-2451

[59] Tan Z, Xie N, Cui H, Moellering DR, Abraham E, Thannickal VJ, et al. Pyruvate dehydrogenase kinase 1 participates in macrophage polarization via regulating glucose metabolism. Journal of Immunology. 2015;**194**(12):6082-6089

[60] Pellegrin M, Bouzourene K, Poitry-Yamate C, Mlynarik V, Feihl F, Aubert JF, et al. Experimental peripheral arterial disease: New insights into muscle glucose uptake, macrophage, and T-cell polarization during early and late stages. Physiological Reports. 2014;**2**(2):e00234

[61] Haschemi A, Kosma P, Gille L, Evans CR, Burant CF, Starkl P, et al. The sedoheptulose kinase CARKL directs macrophage polarization through control of glucose metabolism. Cell Metabolism. 2012;**15**(6):813-826

[62] Ji Y, Sun S, Xu A, Bhargava P, Yang L, Lam KS, et al. Activation of natural killer T cells promotes M2 macrophage polarization in adipose tissue and improves systemic glucose tolerance via interleukin-4 (IL-4)/STAT6 protein signaling axis in obesity. The Journal of Biological Chemistry. 2012;**287**(17):13561-13571

[63] Morey M, O'Gaora P, Pandit A, Helary C. Hyperglycemia acts in synergy with hypoxia to maintain the pro-inflammatory phenotype of macrophages. PLoS One. 2019;**14**(8):e0220577

[64] Pavlou S, Lindsay J, Ingram R, Xu H, Chen M. Sustained high glucose exposure sensitizes macrophage responses to cytokine stimuli but reduces their phagocytic activity. BMC Immunology. 2018;**19**(1):24

[65] Xu F, Zhang C, Graves DT. Abnormal cell responses and role of TNF-alpha in impaired diabetic wound healing. BioMed Research International. 2013;**2013**:754802

[66] Munoz-Garcia J, Cochonneau D, Teletchea S, Moranton E, Lanoe D, Brion R, et al. The twin cytokines interleukin-34 and CSF-1: Masterful conductors of macrophage homeostasis. Theranostics. 2021;**11**(4):1568-1593

[67] Han X, Boisvert WA. Interleukin-10 protects against atherosclerosis by modulating multiple atherogenic macrophage function. Thrombosis and Haemostasis. 2015;**113**(3):505-512

[68] Schmidt DR, Kao WJ. The interrelated role of fibronectin and interleukin-1 in biomaterial-modulated macrophage function. Biomaterials. 2007;**28**(3):371-382

[69] Akira S, Kishimoto T. Role of interleukin-6 in macrophage function. Current Opinion in Hematology. 1996;**3**(1):87-93

[70] Mui AL, Miyajima A. Interleukin-3 and granulocyte-macrophage colony-stimulating factor receptor signal transduction. Proceedings of the Society for Experimental Biology and Medicine. 1994;**206**(3):284-288

[71] Broxmeyer HE. Advances in understanding of biological effects of interleukin-11, leukemia inhibitory factor, and macrophage inflammatory protein 1 alpha. Current Opinion in Hematology. 1994;**1**(3):197-202

[72] Miyajima A, Mui AL, Ogorochi T, Sakamaki K. Receptors for granulocyte-macrophage colony-stimulating factor, interleukin-3, and interleukin-5. Blood. 1993;**82**(7):1960-1974

[73] Aglietta M, Pasquino P, Sanavio F, Stacchini A, Severino A, Fubini L, et al. Granulocyte-macrophage colony stimulating factor and interleukin 3: Target cells and kinetics of response in vivo. Stem Cells. 1993;**11**(Suppl 2):83-87

[74] Lee J, Rodero MP, Patel J, Moi D, Mazzieri R, Khosrotehrani K. Interleukin-23 regulates interleukin-17 expression in wounds, and its inhibition accelerates diabetic wound healing through the alteration of macrophage polarization. The FASEB Journal. 2018;**32**(4):2086-2094

[75] Sharma BR, Kanneganti TD. NLRP3 inflammasome in cancer and metabolic diseases. Nature Immunology. 2021;**22**(5):550-559

[76] Lin TY, Tsai MC, Tu W, Yeh HC, Wang SC, Huang SP, et al. Role of the NLRP3 inflammasome: Insights into cancer hallmarks. Frontiers in Immunology. 2020;**11**:610492

[77] Zhang X, Dai J, Li L, Chen H, Chai Y. NLRP3 Inflammasome expression and Signaling in human diabetic wounds and in high glucose induced macrophages. Journal Diabetes Research. 2017;**2017**:5281358

[78] Amit I, Winter DR, Jung S. The role of the local environment and epigenetics in shaping macrophage identity and their effect on tissue homeostasis. Nature Immunology. 2016;**17**(1):18-25

[79] Barrero MJ, Boue S, Izpisua Belmonte JC. Epigenetic mechanisms that regulate cell identity. Cell Stem Cell. 2010;**7**(5):565-570

[80] Li S, Ding X, Zhang H, Ding Y, Tan Q. IL-25 improves diabetic wound healing through stimulating M2 macrophage polarization and fibroblast activation. International Immunopharmacology. 2022;**106**:108605

[81] Wang N, Wu Y, Zeng N, Wang H, Deng P, Xu Y, et al. E2F1 hinders skin wound healing by repressing vascular endothelial growth factor (VEGF) expression, neovascularization, and macrophage recruitment. PLoS One. 2016;**11**(8):e0160411

[82] Grieb G, Simons D, Eckert L, Hemmrich M, Steffens G, Bernhagen J, et al. Levels of macrophage migration inhibitory factor and glucocorticoids in chronic wound patients and their potential interactions with impaired wound endothelial progenitor cell migration. Wound Repair and Regeneration. 2012;**20**(5):707-714

[83] Li Y, Chen X, Lu C. The interplay between DNA and histone methylation: Molecular mechanisms and disease implications. EMBO Reports. 2021;**22**(5):e51803

[84] Ishii M, Wen H, Corsa CA, Liu T, Coelho AL, Allen RM, et al. Epigenetic regulation of the alternatively activated macrophage phenotype. Blood. 2009;**114**(15):3244-3254

[85] Kimball AS, Davis FM, denDekker A, Joshi AD, Schaller MA, Bermick J, et al. The histone methyltransferase Setdb2 modulates macrophage phenotype and uric acid production in diabetic wound repair. Immunity. 2019;**51**(2):258-271 e255

[86] Kimball AS, Joshi A, Carson WFt, Boniakowski AE, Schaller M, Allen R, Bermick J, Davis FM, Henke PK, Burant CF, Kunkel SL and Gallagher KA. The histone methyltransferase MLL1 directs macrophage-mediated inflammation in wound healing and is altered in a murine model of obesity and type 2 diabetes. Diabetes. 2017;**66**(9):2459-2471

[87] Davis FM, denDekker A, Kimball A, Joshi AD, El Azzouny M, Wolf SJ, et al. Epigenetic regulation of TLR4 in diabetic macrophages modulates Immunometabolism and wound repair. Journal of Immunology. 2020;**204**(9):2503-2513

[88] Davis FM, Kimball A, denDekker A, Joshi AD, Boniakowski AE, Nysz D, et al. Histone methylation directs myeloid TLR4 expression and regulates wound healing following cutaneous tissue injury. Journal of Immunology. 2019;**202**(6):1777-1785

[89] Kittan NA, Allen RM, Dhaliwal A, Cavassani KA, Schaller M, Gallagher KA, et al. Cytokine induced phenotypic and epigenetic signatures are key to establishing specific macrophage phenotypes. PLoS One. 2013;**8**(10):e78045

[90] Davis FM, denDekker A, Joshi AD, Wolf SJ, Audu C, Melvin WJ, et al. Palmitate-TLR4 signaling regulates

the histone demethylase, JMJD3, in macrophages and impairs diabetic wound healing. European Journal of Immunology. 2020;**50**(12): 1929-1940

[91] Takemoto R, Kamiya T, Hara H, Adachi T. Lysyl oxidase expression is regulated by the H3K27 demethylase Jmjd3 in tumor-associated M2-like macrophages. Journal of Clinical Biochemistry and Nutrition. 2020;**66**(2):110-115

[92] Liu S, Wang X, Pan L, Wu W, Yang D, Qin M, et al. Endogenous hydrogen sulfide regulates histone demethylase JMJD3-mediated inflammatory response in LPS-stimulated macrophages and in a mouse model of LPS-induced septic shock. Biochemical Pharmacology. 2018;**149**:153-162

[93] Xuan D, Han Q, Tu Q, Zhang L, Yu L, Murry D, et al. Epigenetic modulation in periodontitis: Interaction of adiponectin and JMJD3-IRF4 axis in macrophages. Journal of Cellular Physiology. 2016;**231**(5):1090-1096

[94] Yan Q, Sun L, Zhu Z, Wang L, Li S, Ye RD. Jmjd3-mediated epigenetic regulation of inflammatory cytokine gene expression in serum amyloid A-stimulated macrophages. Cellular Signalling. 2014;**26**(9):1783-1791

[95] De Santa F, Narang V, Yap ZH, Tusi BK, Burgold T, Austenaa L, et al. Jmjd3 contributes to the control of gene expression in LPS-activated macrophages. The EMBO Journal. 2009;**28**(21):3341-3352

[96] De Santa F, Totaro MG, Prosperini E, Notarbartolo S, Testa G, Natoli G. The histone H3 lysine-27 demethylase Jmjd3 links inflammation to inhibition of polycomb-mediated gene silencing. Cell. 2007;**130**(6):1083-1094

[97] Gallagher KA, Joshi A, Carson WF, Schaller M, Allen R, Mukerjee S, et al. Epigenetic changes in bone marrow progenitor cells influence the inflammatory phenotype and alter wound healing in type 2 diabetes. Diabetes. 2015;**64**(4):1420-1430

[98] Bermick J, Schaller M, Wt C. Histone methylation is critical in monocyte to macrophage differentiation. The FEBS Journal. 2017;**284**(9):1306-1308

[99] Das Gupta K, Shakespear MR, Iyer A, Fairlie DP, Sweet MJ. Histone deacetylases in monocyte/macrophage development, activation and metabolism: Refining HDAC targets for inflammatory and infectious diseases. Clinical & Translational Immunology. 2016;**5**(1):e62

[100] Jiang Y, Fu J, Du J, Luo Z, Guo L, Xu J, et al. DNA methylation alterations and their potential influence on macrophage in periodontitis. Oral Diseases. 2022;**28**(2):249-263

[101] Lentini A, Nestor CE. Mapping DNA methylation in mammals: The state of the art. Methods in Molecular Biology. 2021;**2198**:37-50

[102] Li T, Garcia-Gomez A, Morante-Palacios O, Ciudad L, Ozkaramehmet S, Van Dijck E, et al. SIRT1/2 orchestrate acquisition of DNA methylation and loss of histone H3 activating marks to prevent premature activation of inflammatory genes in macrophages. Nucleic Acids Research. 2020;**48**(2):665-681

[103] Wang X, Cao Q, Yu L, Shi H, Xue B, Shi H. Epigenetic regulation of macrophage polarization and inflammation by DNA methylation in obesity. JCI Insight. 2016;**1**(19):e87748

[104] Yan J, Tie G, Wang S, Tutto A, DeMarco N, Khair L, et al. Diabetes

impairs wound healing by Dnmt1-dependent dysregulation of hematopoietic stem cells differentiation towards macrophages. Nature Communications. 2018;**9**(1):33

[105] Grunstein M. Histone acetylation in chromatin structure and transcription. Nature. 1997;**389**(6649):349-352

[106] Karnam K, Sedmaki K, Sharma P, Routholla G, Goli S, Ghosh B, et al. HDAC6 inhibitor accelerates wound healing by inhibiting tubulin mediated IL-1beta secretion in diabetic mice. Biochimica et Biophysica Acta - Molecular Basis of Disease. 2020;**1866**(11):165903

[107] Cao MX, Jiang YP, Tang YL, Liang XH. The crosstalk between lncRNA and microRNA in cancer metastasis: Orchestrating the epithelial-mesenchymal plasticity. Oncotarget. Feb 14, 2017;**8**(7):12472-12483

[108] Li D, Duan M, Feng Y, Geng L, Li X, Zhang W. MiR-146a modulates macrophage polarization in systemic juvenile idiopathic arthritis by targeting INHBA. Molecular Immunology. 2016;**77**:205-212

[109] Huang C, Liu XJ, QunZhou XJ, Ma TT, Meng XM, Li J. MiR-146a modulates macrophage polarization by inhibiting Notch1 pathway in RAW264.7 macrophages. International Immunopharmacology. 2016;**32**:46-54

[110] O'Connell RM, Taganov KD, Boldin MP, Cheng G, Baltimore D. MicroRNA-155 is induced during the macrophage inflammatory response. Proceedings of the National Academy of Sciences of the United States of America. 2007;**104**(5):1604-1609

[111] Liu M, Meng X, Xuan Z, Chen S, Wang J, Chen Z, et al. Effect of Er Miao San on peritoneal macrophage polarisation through the miRNA-33/NLRP3 signalling pathway in a rat model of adjuvant arthritis. Pharmaceutical Biology. 2022;**60**(1):846-853

[112] Wu S, Xu R, Zhu X, He H, Zhang J, Zeng Q, et al. The long noncoding RNA LINC01140/miR-140-5p/FGF9 axis modulates bladder cancer cell aggressiveness and macrophage M2 polarization. Aging (Albany N Y). 2020;**12**(24):25845-25864

[113] Hu J, Zhang L, Liechty C, Zgheib C, Hodges MM, Liechty KW, et al. Long noncoding RNA GAS5 regulates macrophage polarization and diabetic wound healing. The Journal of Investigative Dermatology. 2020;**140**(8):1629-1638

[114] Tian X, Wu Y, Yang Y, Wang J, Niu M, Gao S, et al. Long noncoding RNA LINC00662 promotes M2 macrophage polarization and hepatocellular carcinoma progression via activating Wnt/beta-catenin signaling. Molecular Oncology. 2020;**14**(2):462-483

[115] Luo H, Zhang Y, Sheng Z, Luo T, Chen J, Liu J, et al. Long noncoding RNA profiling from Fasciola Gigantica excretory/secretory product-induced M2 to M1 macrophage polarization. Cellular Physiology and Biochemistry. 2018;**47**(2):505-522

[116] Ito I, Asai A, Suzuki S, Kobayashi M, Suzuki F. M2b macrophage polarization accompanied with reduction of long noncoding RNA GAS5. Biochemical and Biophysical Research Communications. 2017;**493**(1):170-175

[117] Yan C, Chen J, Yang X, Li W, Mao R, Chen Z. Emerging roles of long non-coding RNAs in diabetic foot ulcers. Diabetes, Metabolic Syndrome and Obesity: Targets and Therapy. 2021;**14**:2549-2560

[118] Karlsson HK, Hallsten K, Bjornholm M, Tsuchida H, Chibalin AV, Virtanen KA, et al. Effects of metformin and rosiglitazone treatment on insulin signaling and glucose uptake in patients with newly diagnosed type 2 diabetes: A randomized controlled study. Diabetes. 2005;**54**(5):1459-1467

[119] Kim SY, Nair MG. Macrophages in wound healing: Activation and plasticity. Immunology and Cell Biology. 2019;**97**(3):258-267

[120] Shen M, Yu H, Jin Y, Mo J, Sui J, Qian X, et al. Metformin facilitates osteoblastic differentiation and M2 macrophage polarization by PI3K/AKT/mTOR pathway in human umbilical cord mesenchymal stem cells. Stem Cells International. 2022;**2022**:9498876

[121] Yuan D, Li Y, Hou L, Yang F, Meng C, Yu Y, et al. Metformin regulates alveolar macrophage polarization to protect against acute lung injury in rats caused by Paraquat poisoning. Frontiers in Pharmacology. 2022;**13**:811372

[122] Xiang X, Zhou L, Lin Z, Qu X, Chen Y, Xia H. Metformin regulates macrophage polarization via the Shh signaling pathway to improve pulmonary vascular development in bronchopulmonary dysplasia. IUBMB Life. 2022;**74**(3):259-271

[123] Qing L, Fu J, Wu P, Zhou Z, Yu F, Tang J. Metformin induces the M2 macrophage polarization to accelerate the wound healing via regulating AMPK/mTOR/NLRP3 inflammasome singling pathway. American Journal of Translational Research. 2019;**11**(2):655-668

[124] Chiang CF, Chao TT, Su YF, Hsu CC, Chien CY, Chiu KC, et al. Metformin-treated cancer cells modulate macrophage polarization through AMPK-NF-kappaB signaling. Oncotarget. 2017;**8**(13):20706-20718

[125] Chen M, Zhang J, Hu F, Liu S, Zhou Z. Metformin affects the features of a human hepatocellular cell line (HepG2) by regulating macrophage polarization in a co-culture microenviroment. Diabetes/Metabolism Research and Reviews. 2015;**31**(8):781-789

[126] Liu W, Yu M, Xie D, Wang L, Ye C, Zhu Q, et al. Melatonin-stimulated MSC-derived exosomes improve diabetic wound healing through regulating macrophage M1 and M2 polarization by targeting the PTEN/AKT pathway. Stem Cell Research & Therapy. 2020;**11**(1):259

[127] Moore K, Thomas A, Harding KG. Iodine released from the wound dressing Iodosorb modulates the secretion of cytokines by human macrophages responding to bacterial lipopolysaccharide. The International Journal of Biochemistry & Cell Biology. 1997;**29**(1):163-171

[128] Das A, Abas M, Biswas N, Banerjee P, Ghosh N, Rawat A, et al. A modified collagen dressing induces transition of inflammatory to reparative phenotype of wound macrophages. Scientific Reports. 2019;**9**(1):14293

[129] Takeuchi T, Ito M, Yamaguchi S, Watanabe S, Honda M, Imahashi T, et al. Hydrocolloid dressing improves wound healing by increasing M2 macrophage polarization in mice with diabetes. Nagoya Journal of Medical Science. 2020;**82**(3):487-498

[130] Das A, Datta S, Roche E, Chaffee S, Jose E, Shi L, et al. Novel mechanisms of collagenase Santyl ointment (CSO) in wound macrophage polarization and resolution of wound inflammation. Scientific Reports. 2018;**8**(1):1696

[131] Aytac A, Demir CI, Alagoz MS. Docosahexaenoic acid improves diabetic

wound healing in a rat model by restoring impaired plasticity of macrophage progenitor cells. Plastic and Reconstructive Surgery. 2021;**148**(5):848e-849e

[132] Strong AL, Levi B. Discussion: Docosahexaenoic acid improves diabetic wound healing in a rat model by restoring impaired plasticity of macrophage progenitor cells. Plastic and Reconstructive Surgery. 2020;**145**(5):951e-952e

[133] Ahmed R, Afreen A, Tariq M, Zahid AA, Masoud MS, Ahmed M, et al. Bone marrow mesenchymal stem cells preconditioned with nitric-oxide-releasing chitosan/PVA hydrogel accelerate diabetic wound healing in rabbits. Biomedical Materials. 2021;**16**(3) [Online ahead of print]

[134] Yang HY, Fierro F, So M, Yoon DJ, Nguyen AV, Gallegos A, et al. Combination product of dermal matrix, human mesenchymal stem cells, and timolol promotes diabetic wound healing in mice. Stem Cells Translational Medicine. 2020;**9**(11):1353-1364

[135] Guo J, Hu H, Gorecka J, Bai H, He H, Assi R, et al. Adipose-derived mesenchymal stem cells accelerate diabetic wound healing in a similar fashion as bone marrow-derived cells. American Journal of Physiology. Cell Physiology. 2018;**315**(6):C885-C896

[136] Zhu L, Wang G, Fischbach S, Xiao X. Suppression of microRNA-205-5p in human mesenchymal stem cells improves their therapeutic potential in treating diabetic foot disease. Oncotarget. 2017;**8**(32):52294-52303

[137] Zhu L, Zhong Q, Yang T, Xiao X. Improved therapeutic effects on diabetic foot by human mesenchymal stem cells expressing MALAT1 as a sponge for microRNA-205-5p. Aging (Albany N Y). 2019;**11**(24):12236-12245

[138] Jiang Y, Chen A, Kline D, Liu Q, Ma J, Wang Y, et al. Polarized macrophages promote gestational beta cell growth through extracellular signal-regulated kinase 5 signalling. Diabetes, Obesity & Metabolism. Sep 2022;**24**(9):1721-1733

[139] Zhu L, Qian J, Jiang Y, Yang T, Duan Q, Xiao X. PlGF reduction compromises angiogenesis in diabetic foot disease through macrophages. Frontiers in Immunology. 2021;**12**:736153

[140] Chen Z, Fu S, Wu Z, Chen J, Huang Y, Wang Y, et al. Relationship between plasma angiogenic growth factors and diabetic foot ulcers. Clinica Chimica Acta. 2018;**482**:95-100

Chapter 4

Tendon Balancing for Diabetic Foot Ulcers, Foot Pain and Charcot Foot

James Monroe Laborde

Abstract

Diabetes mellitus causes patients to develop sensory and motor neuropathy. Sensory neuropathy in patients with diabetes results in decrease in protective sensation. Motor neuropathy causes tendon imbalance. Tendon imbalance causes increased mechanical stress in the foot. This increased stress can cause foot pain and calluses and can progress to forefoot ulcers. Less often the ligaments fail before the skin, which can cause arch collapse and then a midfoot ulcer of Charcot foot. Foot pain in diabetics is common and frequently results from Achilles tendinitis, plantar fasciitis, midfoot arthritis and metatarsalgia. Tendon balancing can decrease stress in the foot which can relieve foot pain, heal forefoot and midfoot ulcers, prevent ulcer recurrence, and prevent progression of deformity in Charcot foot. Tendon balancing could prevent most of the amputations now being done on diabetic patients. Tendon balancing should be used earlier and more often in treatment of diabetic foot ulcers, foot pain and Charcot foot.

Keywords: diabetic foot ulcers, foot pain, Charcot foot, diabetes

1. Introduction

Patients with diabetic neuropathy develop foot problems, some of which can improve with surgery. Tendon balancing is one of the procedures used to treat diabetic foot problems. Tendon lengthening, such as gastrocnemius-soleus recession (GSR), has fewer complications than bony procedures in the foot [1–6].

Tendon lengthening should be performed before bony procedures in high-risk patients such as diabetics, patients with foot ulcers, infection, smokers and without pedal pulses [1–6]. Imbalance of tendons, especially Achilles tightness, can aggravated or cause or many foot problems [1–7]. Tendon lengthening can be used as part of treatment for many foot problems [2, 7–12].

A large number of patients have diabetes and the number is increasing [13]. Foot ulcers are common in patients with diabetes mellitus [14, 15]. Foot ulcers can lead to infection and amputation. Amputation can result from infection from foot ulcers [15, 16]. Over 80% of amputations in diabetic patients have foot ulcers [15, 16].

The most common chronic wounds in industrialized countries are foot ulcers [17, 18]. The average excess cost of a foot ulcer over a two-year period is over $25,000 [19].

The most common reason for diabetic patient to be admitted to the hospital is foot infection [20]. Up to 50% (62/133) amputation and 20% (26/133) major amputation can occur in patients admitted for foot ulcer or foot infection [16]. Over 80,000 amputations have occurred in diabetic patients in the U.S in one year [21]. If foot ulcers could be cured, most amputations in diabetics could potentially be prevented [15, 16].

The most common cause of neuropathy is diabetes mellitus [22, 23]. Neuropathy causes decreased protective sensation and motor neuropathy causes tendon tightness [24–26]. Tightness of tendon, especially the Achilles, causes increased forces in the foot [27]. Increased forces in the forefoot can cause a callus followed by a forefoot ulcer [14, 27]. Increased forces in the foot can also cause Charcot foot, including foot arthritis, arch collapse, midfoot bony prominence and then midfoot ulcer [10, 28]. Foot ulcers can also result from other causes of neuropathy besides diabetes and can be treated in the same way [24, 26, 29].

2. Foot ulcer treatment

Foot ulcers are of managed by addressing infection, arterial disease and high forces in the foot. Infection is treated with antibiotics and debridement. Which antibiotic is determined by deep culture and, if needed, infectious disease consultation [30]. Vascular evaluation and treatment is recommended if the patient lacks both pedal pulses. Hyperbaric oxygen may a decrease the frequency of major amputations, but more studies are needed to confirm its causation in the decrease [31].

Off-loading consists of decreasing force in the foot. Forces in the foot can be decreased by tendon lengthening [27]. More ulcers than wound care and total contact casting (TCC) are healed by tendon lengthening [2, 24–26, 29, 32–39]. Tendon lengthening treatment of foot ulcers has good literature support [2, 24–27, 29, 33–41].

TCC, walking boots, and modified shoes helps heal foot ulcers [14]. However, TCC are difficult to apply, and has a higher complication rate and higher rate of recurrent ulceration than does tendon lengthening [32, 33]. Tendon lengthening removal of prominent metatarsal heads have similar results similar but with more transfer ulcers when only metatarsal head is removed [3].

3. Results of foot ulcers treatment

3.1 Tendon lengthening

Multiple authors reported the association of gastrocnemius-soleus contracture, neuropathy, and chronic ulceration of the forefoot [24–26]. The high rate of successful healing of forefoot ulcers after Achilles lengthening was reported in multiple studies [24–26, 33–36, 41]. Also a high rate of healing of midfoot and toe ulcers also occurred after tendon lengthening [2, 29].

The recurrence rate of foot ulcers after three years in diabetic patients treated without tendon lengthening, was 61% (286/468) [42]. After Achilles tendon lengthening, forefoot ulcer recurrence rates were much lower, 14% [41]. There is also a low rate of recurrence of toe ulcers treated with toe flexor tenotomy and with midfoot ulcers treated with tendon lengthening [2, 29].

Mueller et al. reported recurrence 10 of 26 ulcers 2 years after Achilles lengthening [33]. Adding peroneus longus and posterior tibial to gastrocnemius–soleus recession (GSR) yielded less recurrence, 3 of 18 at 45 months follow-up [26]. Dayer and Assal also had a low recurrence (1/22) by adding tendon procedures such as peroneus longus transfer to gastrocnemius recession [36].

The intention of tendon lengthening is to decrease force on the area of ulceration. The pressure on the first metatarsal head should decrease with peroneus longus lengthening as the pressure on the fifth metatarsal should be decreased with posterior tibial lengthening. Force on the entire plantar forefoot should decrease with GSR. Armstrong et al. demonstrated that Achilles lengthening does in fact decrease pressure on the forefoot and recommended this procedure to help treat and prevent foot ulceration [27].

Multiple authors lengthened the Achilles tendon by Hoke's method of hemisection at 3 levels of the tendon [25, 33, 35]. Holstein warned that Hoke's procedure for diabetic forefoot ulcers caused 7/75 Achilles ruptures and 11/75 heel ulcers in his patients [35]. Achilles tenectomy for distal ulcers after transmetatarsal amputation had 4/32 (13%) plantar heel ulcers [34]. Subcutaneous tenotomy method of Strohmeyer was used by Yospovitch and Sheskin [24, 43]. Vulpius technique of GSR is used by this author [44]. A very low rate of heel ulcers and other complications of GSR has been reported [2, 26, 36, 41].

Takahashi and Shrestha used the Vulpius procedure successfully to correct Achilles tightness in 230 adults after cerebrovascular accident [1]. Ninety-eight were diabetics and the average age was 68 and had no tendon or incision problems.

The results appear to be good whatever technique of lengthening of the gastrocnemius-soleus or Achilles tendon, [41]. Choice of the surgeon can determine the technique of Achilles lengthening for forefoot ulcers.

Tendon lengthening literature shows better results than other treatments for forefoot and midfoot ulcers [41]. Tendon lengthening should be used more often to treat of diabetic ulcers forefoot and midfoot ulcers [2, 24–26, 29, 33–37, 40, 41].

3.2 Wound care and Total contact casting (TCC)

TCC resulted in healing in 90% (64/71) of foot ulcers [45]. However ulcer recurrence at 18 months follow-up occurred in 34% (22/64). A high complication rate of 31% (22/70) has also been reported with TCC [32]. A comparison of healed ulcers at two year follow-up revealed 81% (21/26) recurred after TCC but only 38% (10/ 27) recurred after Achilles lengthening was added in the only controlled randomized study available [33].

TCC is apparently not needed for forefoot ulcer healing, since TCC was not used in most more recent studies after Mueller's article [26, 29, 33, 35, 41]. Wound care healed only 31% (142/458) of diabetic foot ulcers in 5 months in a meta-analysis of the literature [38]. An average of 80% of diabetic foot ulcers healed with TCC [39]. Tendon lengthening has better healing rate for ulcers than wound care and TCC [2, 24–26, 29, 33–36, 38–41].

Tendon lengthening also has less complications and a much lower recurrence rate than TCC [2, 24–26, 29, 32–36, 41]. This author agrees with other authors that tendon lengthening rather than TCC should be considered the "gold standard" treatment for forefoot ulcers [26, 36, 41].

3.3 Metatarsal head removal

Foot surgeons have recommended metatarsal head resection to heal ulcers plantar to metatarsal heads. Even though this procedure frequently resulted in ulcer healing, transfer metatarsal ulcer frequently occurred later. Transfer ulcers occurred in 52% (53/101) of patients in the 35 months of follow-up after metatarsal head resection [3].

Repeated transfer ulcer and metatarsal head removal can result in gradual resection of the forefoot, then amputation stump ulcer and possible major amputation [42].

Tendon lengthening can be used instead of metatarsal head resection to decrease the potential for transfer ulcers resulting from the increased pressure on the forefoot. The metatarsal head should be removed if bone infection is severe enough to cause bone fragmentation or necrotic tissue. The metatarsal head can be removed if osteomyelitis persists after the ulcer healing and antibiotics completion [26].

3.4 Osteotomy of metatarsal

A high rate, 95% (21/22), of successful healing of neuropathic forefoot ulcers occurred after dorsiflexion metatarsal osteotomy [4]. However, a 68% complication rate occurred with seven patients developing acute Charcot disease, three developing midfoot ulcers, three deep wound infections, two transfer ulcers under adjacent metatarsal heads, and one transtibial amputation. Fewer complications occurred after tendon lengthening for forefoot ulcers resulted with no new or worsening Charcot arthritis or foot arthritis, new mid-foot ulcers, transfer metatarsal ulcers or wound infections [26]. After tendon lengthening complication rate is less than after metatarsal osteotomy and similar to non-operative treatment [4, 16, 26].

3.5 Amputation

Amputation becomes necessary when infection and gangrene progress. In one study of amputations in diabetic patients, 84% (67/80) were attributed to foot ulcers [16]. In diabetics with forefoot ulcers, ray amputation resulted in transfer ulcers occurred in 12% (11/89) and additional amputation in 18% (16/89) [46]. Transmetatarsal amputation has used to treat chronic diabetic forefoot ulcers [47]. This resulted in wound breakdown in 9% (8/85), transtibial amputation in 26% (17/65) and 30% (17/57) death. Tendon lengthening complication rates lower than above have been reported with for forefoot ulcers [26, 41]. To increase healing rate to 81%, Pinzur et al. recommended Achilles lengthening be done at same time as transmetatarsal amputation (52/64) [48]. Achilles tenotomy was recommended by Lieberman et al. with midfoot (Chopart) amputation for gangrene and/or infection [49]. For forefoot ulcers, tendon lengthening seems to be better than amputation. Also combining Achilles lengthening with ray or transmetatarsal amputation for forefoot gangrene and/or severe infection appears preferable. By putting glove over infected foot, doing tendon lengthening first, applying dressing to leg, removing glove and then preforming partial foot amputation, tendon lengthening can be done at time of amputation without infection of proximal incisions.

The reported amputation rate was 16% (80/514) and 17% (78/468) during three years after healing of foot ulcers, [23, 42]. No patients (0/16) required amputation for progressive infection at average follow-up of 45 months in one study of tendon lengthening for forefoot ulcers [26]. More proximal major amputation may become necessary when all other treatments fail.

4. Vascular disease

Gangrene in diabetics is primarily vascular problem. Arterial disease can aggravate most other diabetic foot problems. Vascular evaluation is recommended in patients without pedal pulses. Patients with palpable dorsalis pedis or posterior tibial arteries require no additional studies. Arterial Doppler is recommend for patients without both of those pedal pulses. Ankle-brachial index (ABI) has been used by others for lower extremity arterial evaluation. The ABI is calculated by dividing systolic pressure at the ankle by that at the arm. An abnormal ABI is 0.90 or below [50]. Vascular surgery evaluation should be obtained If the Doppler study shows near or complete blockage or if ABI is abnormal.

Vascular disease has been considered to be a contraindication to TCC [45]. Foot ulcers in patients without both pedal pulses can be salvageable with tendon lengthening [26, 29, 31].

5. Tendon lengthening treatment

Patients with foot ulcers can be considered for tendon lengthening after vascular and infection have been treated. Diabetes mellitus and vascular disease are the most common co-morbidities with neuropathic foot problems [26, 29]. These patients frequently have complications. Tendon lengthening has less complications than bony procedures [1–6, 26, 29, 41]. Soft tissue procedures are usually performed first since they have lower complication rates, and then if they fail, bony procedures are done later.

Level I and level III studies have only been done for metatarsal head ulcers [25, 33, 36]. JBJS instructions for authors explains levels of evidence. There are however many level IV studies demonstrating effectiveness of tendon lengthening for foot ulcers [24, 26, 29, 34, 35, 41]. Level IV studies have advantages that the study populations are more likely to be representative of the population of interest, results are closer to those obtained in clinical practice, have a higher relevance and external validity and can be better applied to clinical practice [51]. Tendon lengthenings as the treatment of choice for diabetic forefoot ulcers seems to be supported by the above studies.

5.1 Metatarsal head forefoot ulcers

If infection is present, patients with ulcers are treated with antibiotics then debridement and tendon lengthening [26]. The foot is covered with a sterile glove after the patient's skin is prepped in the operating room. Calf and ankle level tendon lengthening is done first and dressing applied. Glove is then removed for debridement of the foot and lengthening of toe tendons if needed. If gangrene of forefoot is present, debridement of gangrenous tissue and GSR are done to decrease pressure on the forefoot and to aid wound healing [41, 46, 48]. Vascular evaluation and wound care are also suggested. If forefoot wound healing is delayed after only debridement, transmetatarsal amputation [34], or Charcot arthropathy with or without ulcer [2], they are offered GSR. If gangrene of midfoot and/or hindfoot is present, transtibial or transfemoral amputation is suggested. Achilles lengthening to prevent ulcers is recommended for progressive metatarsal calluses [27].

GSR is used to treat all patients with ulcers plantar to metatarsal heads [24–26, 33, 35, 41]. With the patient supine the surgery is performed, while the knee is flexed and externally rotated. A stack of towels is placed under foot with the surgeon is seated on the opposite side. Vulpius technique [1, 26] is used, transecting the gastrocnemius tendon and underlying aponeurosis of the soleus just distal to the gastrocnemius muscle [44]. Ankle is dorsiflexed to 20–30°. Staples are used to close midcalf posterior longitudinal incision 5 cm. long after 3–0 absorbable suture closes the subcuticular layer. For recurrent ulcers and if patient can only tolerate local anesthesia percutaneous triple cut Achilles tenotomy can be used.

For first metatarsal ulcers peroneus longus (Z-type) lengthening is combined with GSR [26]. Incision is proximal to the ankle joint. The tendon repair is done with a 2–0 absorbable suture with no tension, with the first metatarsal is in maximum dorsiflexion and the foot is in maximum inversion. For fifth metatarsal ulcers posterior tibial lengthening is also performed [26]. Z-type lengthening is also performed through medial incision 5–10 cm. proximal to the ankle joint. Same technique is used to close these incisions. Repeat GSR or triple cut Achilles lengthening and percutaneous metatarsal osteotomy for recurrent metatarsal ulcers.

Full weight bearing is allowed immediately in a walking boot, which is worn for four to six weeks. Crutches or a walker is offered to the patient if needed for balance when surgery is bilateral. Ulcer treatment is clean dressings changed weekly. Skin staples are removed at two weeks. Diabetic-type shoes are recommended after six weeks. Double heel lift exercises are begun at 2 months and at 3 months single heel lift exercises. They can resume standing all day at work at 3 months. Running, jumping and climbing are allowed at 6 months.

5.2 Toe ulcer treatment

Percutaneous toe flexor tenotomy at the proximal portion of the proximal phalanx is used for plantar toe ulcers [29, 52]. This can be done in the office, but can be done in the operating room if the patient is there for some other reason. Alcohol is used to prepare the toe, and then local anesthetic is given. Toe is extended so the tendons are palpable. Through a small (2 mm) transverse incision, both flexor tendons are transected. A sudden increase in extension of the distal and proximal interphalangeal joints of the lesser toes confirms division of both flexor tendons. After the flexor hallucis longus (FHL) is divided a sudden increase in extension of the interphalangeal joint of the hallux occurs. Suture is not used unless bleeding is excessive but incision is covered with sterile gauze. A postoperative shoe, sandal or extra-depth shoe can be used. Patients are allowed full weight-bearing. Patients return weekly until the ulcer heals.

Percutaneous extensor and flexor tenotomy can be used for a dorsal ulcer of PIP joint. Percutaneous capsulotomy dorsal metatarsal-phalangeal (MP) and volar (PIP) are also performed if needed. Percutaneous phalangeal osteotomy is performed if correction is insufficient.

For interdigital ulcers of the first web space, patients are offered percutaneous adductor tenotomy, and lateral capsule release of the first MP joint. An interdigital ulcer of the lessor toes may also have percutaneous MP capsular release in the lessor toe in addition to first toe surgery. Percutaneous phalangeal osteotomy or removal of prominent bone is performed if ulcer persists or recurs. Toe amputation is usually performed for osteomyelitis in the toe which is not controlled with antibiotics.

5.3 Charcot foot

Midfoot ulcers can develop plantar to the bony prominence in the area of arch collapse from Charcot neuropathic arthropathy (Charcot foot). Exostectomy or fusion have recommended to be combined with Achilles lengthening [53–56]. Good preliminary results have been found with tendon lengthening (GSR) alone as the initial treatment for midfoot ulcers: 9/10 ulcers healed, 1/9 recurred with less complications than bony procedures [2, 5, 6]. Tendon lengthening (GSR) seems to heal these ulcers, prevent progression of bony deformity and promote consolidation of fragmented midfoot bone [2, 57]. The lack of progression of deformity and low recurrence rate of GSR also compare favorably with the 41/140 (36%) deformity progression and 43/140 (37%) ulceration after non-operative treatment [56, 57].

Removal of plantar bony prominence percutaneously with a burr is now routinely added to GSR. Posterior tibial lengthening can be added for lateral midfoot ulcers and peroneal tendon lengthening for medial midfoot ulcers. GSR results in much fewer heel ulcers than does Achilles tendon lengthening [1, 41, 58, 59]. If the ulcer fails to heal or recurs, then tendon lengthening and percutaneous removal of the midfoot bony prominence (exostectomy) can be repeated [5, 41]. If the ulcer fails to heal or recurs, if there is no bony prominence and the foot is unstable, then midfoot fusion can be performed [6]. Soft tissue surgery is advantageous because diabetic patients have a higher complication rate with foot and ankle surgery [60].

Lengthening the Achilles in Charcot arthropathy was recommended by Thomas and Huffman [55]. Tendon lengthening is recommended for early stage Charcot foot to relieve pain, promote consolidation, prevent progression of deformity and heal or prevent midfoot ulceration from arch collapse [2, 57]. Bony procedures are less commonly done if tendon lengthening fails. Amputation is kept as a last resort.

5.4 Results of tendon lengthening

A 47% decrease in major amputations in Medicare patients with diabetic foot ulcers between 2000 and 2010 has been reported [61]. In the same period Achilles tendon lengthening increased 89% and gastrocnemius recession increased 575%. The authors felt the main cause of decrease in major amputations was the increase in tendon lengthening. Recently performed a literature review on diabetic foot ulcer treatment and gave the highest recommendation (supported by strong evidence) to tendon lengthening [62].

Available evidence seems to indicate that tendon lengthening is the most effective treatment for plantar diabetic foot ulcers with the least complications [41, 57]. Tendon lengthening can also relieve foot pain, prevent ulcers and Charcot foot, and stop progression of Charcot arch collapse to rocker bottom foot, midfoot ulceration and amputation [57, 63]. Tendon lengthening may be combined with other modalities but should be done as soon as possible to promote rapid healing before the ulcer gets infected and to better prevent new, recurrent and transfer ulcers, progression of deformity and amputation [41, 57].

Yammine and Assi noted underuse of tendon lengthening which offered excellent outcomes with more ulcers healed faster with less recurrence, transfer ulcers, infection and amputation than nonsurgical treatment [64, 65]. This author recommends tendon lengthening as part of initial treatment for diabetic plantar forefoot and midfoot ulcers and Charcot of the midfoot [41, 57].

6. Pain in foot

Diabetic patients without ulcers tend to have less neuropathy. They frequently develop painful foot problems including Achilles tendinitis, plantar fasciitis, foot arthritis and metatarsalgia.

McGlamery and Kitting stated that tight Achilles is the underlying cause of most foot problems and that permanent correction is only achieved by correction of Achilles tightness [7]. Achilles tightness is common in patients with Charcot foot, plantar fasciitis, Achilles tendinitis, metatarsalgia, foot arthritis, Morton's neuroma and hallux valgus [66, 67].

Gastrocnemius recession (GR) has been recommended for the treatment of these problems in patients without neuropathy or diabetes [8–12, 68]. Anderson et al. felt that gastrocnemius tightness causes metatarsalgia, plantar fasciitis, Achilles tendinitis and arch pain [10, 68]. Achilles tightness, can cause progressive arch collapse, foot arthritis and flat foot which can progress to posterior tibial tendon dysfunction and heel valgus. High (94%, 32/34) patient satisfaction has been reported using GSR for plantar fasciitis. Anderson felt GR not only helped the pain of these conditions but prevents the progression described above [10, 68]. Several authors recommend GR for pain relief in patients with arch collapse, foot and ankle arthritis, Achilles tendinitis, plantar fasciitis, posterior tibial tendinitis [8–12, 68]. GR may be useful in preventing these problems and foot ulcers so is especially useful in diabetic patients [10, 27].

7. Other toe problems

Painful hammer, mallet or claw toes, especially with progressive toe callus, are offered toe flexor tenotomy after failure of non-operative treatment. These procedures are also done both for pain relief and to help prevent future ulcers in diabetic patients. Percutaneous capsulotomy and/or percutaneous phalangeal osteotomy are performed if correction is insufficient. Percutaneous interphalangeal joint resection and fusion is less commonly performed. Percutaneous pins are used as needed and removed at 3 weeks.

For interdigital corns of the first web space, patients are offered percutaneous shaving of bone under corn and adductor tenotomy of first metatarsal-phalangeal (MP) joint. Interdigital corns of lessor toes may have percutaneous shaving of bone under corn and capsular release in the lessor toe MP joint in addition if needed.

Inactive high-risk patients with painful arthritis of the first MP joint can be treated initially with percutaneous FHL tenotomy to relieve pain and prevent ulceration with less expected complications than with bone surgery [69]. More commonly, percutaneous resection of bone spurs, dorsal MP joint (cheilectomy)and proximal phalangeal dorsal closing wedge osteotomy is performed [70]. DePrado's book on percutaneous is an excellent "how to" book on percutaneous foot surgery [70].

For bunions, percutaneous or open chevron metatarsal osteotomy and proximal phalanx osteotomy are performed [70, 71]. Most patients having first ray surgery for arthritis or bunions also have GSR for Achilles tightness. If they have diabetes, GSR will more likely relieve their pain and prevent foot ulcers, Charcot foot and amputation [41, 57]. If they have Achilles tendinitis, posterior tibial tendinitis or dysfunction, midfoot arthritis or metatarsalgia in addition to their first MP pain, they are more likely to have their pain relieved than if they have bunionectomy alone [41, 68].

8. Additional studies

Additional studies should be done in diabetics to see if frequent eccentric calf stretching can prevent calf tightness, forefoot calluses, forefoot ulceration and

Charcot arthritis. Since calf stretching would not harm diabetic patients, this author recommends prophylactic eccentric calf stretching to these patients.

Achilles tendon lengthening has been recommended to prevent re-ulceration in patients with prior ulcers [27]. More studies are needed to confirm tendon lengthening is helpful in preventing ulceration in patients with progressive callus, prior ulcers, and impending ulcers [27] and whether tendon lengthening should be used as part of primary initial treatment for foot ulcers and Charcot foot [41, 57].

Thomas and Huffman recommended lengthening the Achilles in Charcot foot [55]. More studies should also be done to confirm that tendon lengthening heals most midfoot ulcers [2], transmetatarsal stump ulcers [34], and ischemic wounds of forefoot [48, 49]. Further studies are also needed to confirm tendon lengthening prevents Charcot foot, prevents progression of deformity of Charcot arthritis of the midfoot [2, 10] and ankle, and prevents foot ulcers and amputation in patients with Charcot foot [57].

Preliminary results of tendon lengthening have been encouraging; however, further studies need to be done to confirm tendon lengthening relieves foot pain from multiple causes and prevents foot ulcers, arch collapse, arthritis, amputation and other foot problems.

9. Conclusions

The literature indicates that tendon lengthening is effective treatment for neuropathic forefoot ulcerations and that the complication rate seems to be low. By healing most forefoot ulcerations and lowering their recurrence rate more than all other treatments, this procedure should lower the incidence of progression of metatarsal ulceration to infection and subsequent amputation. More studies need to be done to confirm tendon lengthening is an effective treatment for Charcot foot and other foot problems and confirm tendon lengthening should be part of initial treatment of diabetic foot problems.

Conflict of interest

The author declares no conflict of interest.

Author details

James Monroe Laborde
Louisiana State University Health Science Center, New Orleans, LA, USA

*Address all correspondence to: monroe@laborde.net

References

[1] Takahashi S, Shrestha A. The Vulpius procedure for correction of equinus deformity in patients with hemiplegia. Journal of Bone and Joint Surgery. 2002;**84B**(7):978-980

[2] Laborde JM. Midfoot ulcers treated with tendon lengthenings. Foot & Ankle International. 2009;**30**(9):842-846

[3] Weiman TJ, Mercke YK, Cerrito PB, Taber SW. Resection of the metatarsal head for diabetic foot ulcers. American Journal of Surgery. 1998;**176**:436-441

[4] Fleischli JE, Anderson RB, Davis WH. Dorsiflexion metatarsal osteotomy for treatment of recalcitrant diabetic neuropathic ulcers. Foot & Ankle International. 1999;**20**(2):80-85

[5] Weiman TJ, Griffiths GD, Polk HC. Management of diabetic midfoot ulcers. Annals of Surgery. 1992;**215**(6):627-630

[6] Early JS, Hansen ST. Surgical reconstruction of the diabetic foot: A salvage approach for midfoot collapse. Foot & Ankle International. 1996;**17**(60):325-330

[7] McGlamary ED, Kitting RW. Equinus foot. Journal of the American Podiatric Medical Association. 1973;**63**(5):165-184

[8] Trepman E, Lutter LD, Richardson EG, Thordavson DB, Gill LH, Digiovanni CR. Special report: Highlights of the 23rd annual summer meeting of the American Orthopaedic Foot and Ankle Society. 2007. Foot & Ankle International. 2008;**29**(1):105-110

[9] Anderson JG, Maskill D, Bohay DR, Conaway D. Gastrocnemius recession: Effective remedy for recalcitrant foot pain. AAOS Now. 2007;**Oct**:10

[10] Anderson JG. Gastrocnemius recession to treat isolated foot pain. In: American Orthopaedic Foot & Ankle Society, 38th Annual Winter Meeting Program. Rosemont, IL: American Orthopedic Foot & Ankle Society; 2008. pp. 90-95

[11] Digovanni CW, Roderick K, Tejwani N, Price R, Hansen ST, Cziernecki J, et al. Isolated gastrocnemius tightness. JBJS. 2002;**84**(6):962-970

[12] Gentchos CE, Bohay DR, Anderson JR. Gastrocnemius recession as treatment for refractory Achilles tendinopathy. Foot & Ankle International. 2008;**29**(6):620-623

[13] National Diabetes Information Clearinghouse (NDIC) NIH Publication No. 06-3892. National Institutes of Health: Bethesda, MD; 2005. Available from: http://diabetes.niddk.nih.gov/dm/pubs/statistics/index.htm

[14] Kahn R. American diabetes association consensus development conference on diabetic foot wound care. Diabetes Care. 1999;**22**(8):1354-1360

[15] Reiber GE, Boyko EJ, Smith DG. Lower extremity foot ulcers and amputations in diabetics. In: Harris MI, Cowie CC, Stern MP, Boyko EJ, Reiber GE, Bennett PH, editors. Diabetes in America. 2nd ed. Washington, DC: US Government Printing Office; 1995 (HDDS pub. No. 95-1468). pp. 408-428

[16] Pecoraro RE, Reiber GE, Burgess EM. Pathways to diabetic limb amputation. Diabetes Care. 1990;**13**(5):213-221

[17] Hosalker HS, Reddy S, Mariani C, Keenan MA. What's new in orthopaedic

rehabilitation. Journal of Bone and Joint Surgery. 2007;**89A**(10):2321

[18] Edelman D. An evidence-based approach to foot ulcer prevention in patients with diabetes. Journal of Clinical Outcomes Management. 1999;**6**:35-40

[19] Ramsey SD, Newton K, Blough D, et al. Incidence outcomes and costs of foot ulcers in patients with diabetes. Diabetes Care. 1999;**22**:382-387

[20] Pinzur MS, Slovenkai MP, Trepman E, Shields NN. Guidelines for diabetic foot care: Recommendations endorsed by the diabetes committee of the American Orthopaedic Foot and Ankle Society. Foot & Ankle International. 2005;**26**(1):113-119

[21] Center for Disease Control, Department of Health and Human Services, National Diabetes Fact Sheet. 2005. Available from: www.cdc.gov/diabetes

[22] Van der Ven A, Chapman CB, Bowker JH. Charcot neuropathy of the foot & ankle. Journal of the American Academy of Orthopaedic Surgeons. 2009;**17**(9):562-571

[23] Young MJ, Boulton AJ, MacLeod AF, Williams DR, Sonksen PH. A multicenter study of the prevalence of diabetic peripheral neuropathy in the United Kingdom hospital clinic population. Diabetologia. 1993;**96**(2):150-154

[24] Yosipovitch Z, Sheskin J. Subcutaneous Achilles tenotomy in the treatment of perforating ulcer of the foot in leprosy. International Journal of Leprosy and Other Mycobacterial Diseases. 1971;**39**:631-632

[25] Lin SS, Lee H, Wapner KL. Plantar forefoot ulceration with equinus deformity of the ankle in diabetic patients; the effect of tendo-Achilles lengthening and total contact casting. Orthopaedics. 1996;**19**(5):465-474

[26] Laborde JM. Neuropathic plantar forefoot ulcers treated with tendon lengthening. Foot & Ankle International. 2008;**24**(4):378-384

[27] Armstrong DG, Shea SS, Nguyen H, Harkless LB. Lengthening of the Achilles tendon in diabetic patients who are at high risk for ulceration of the foot. Journal of Bone and Joint Surgery. 1999;**81-A**(4):535-538

[28] Pinzur MS. Current concepts review: Charcot arthropathy of the foot and ankle. Foot & Ankle International. 2007;**28**(8):952-959

[29] Laborde JM. Neuropathic toe ulcers treated with flexor tenotomies. Foot & Ankle International. 2007;**28**(11):1160-1164

[30] Bader MS. Diabetic foot infection. American Family Physician. 2008;**78**(1):71-79.31

[31] Hinchliffe RJ, ValkGD ADG, Armstrong DG, Bakker K, Game FL, Hartemann-Heurtier A, et al. A systematic review of the effectiveness of interventions to enhance the healing of chronic ulcers of the foot in diabetes. Diabetes/Metabolism Research and Reviews. 2008;**24**(S1):119-144

[32] Guyton GP. An analysis of iatrogenic complications of total contact cast. Foot & Ankle International. 2005;**26**(11):903-907

[33] Mueller MJ, Sinacore DR, Hastings MK, Strube MJ, Johnson JE. Effect of Achilles tendon lengthening on neuropathic plantar ulcers, a randomized clinical trial. Journal of Bone and Joint Surgery. 2003;**85A**(8):1436-1445

[34] Barry DC, Sabacinski KA, Habershaw GM, Giurin JM, Chrzan JS. Tendo Achilles procedure for chronic ulceration in diabetic patients with transmetatarsal amputations. Journal of the American Podiatric Medical Association. 1993;**83**(2):96-100

[35] Holstein P, Lohman M, Birtsch M, Jorgensen B. Achilles tendon lengthening, the panacea for plantar forefoot ulcers? Diabetes/Metabolism Research and Reviews. 2004;**20**(S1):S37-S40

[36] Dayer R, Assal M. Chronic diabetic ulcers under the first metatarsal head treated by staged tendon balancing. JBJS. 2009;**91B**(4):487-493

[37] Nishimoto GS, Attinger CE, Cooper PS. Lengthening the Achilles tendon for the treatment of diabetic plantar forefoot ulceration. Surgical Clinics of North America. 2003;**83**:707-726

[38] Margolis DJ, Kantor J, Berlin JA. Healing of diabetic neuropathic foot ulcers receiving standard treatment. Diabetes Care. 1999;**22**(5):692-695

[39] Apelqvist J, Larsson J, Agarth CD. Long-term prognosis for diabetic patients with foot ulcers. Journal of Internal Medicine. 1993;**233**(6):485-491

[40] Strauss MB. The orthopaedic surgeon's role in the treatment and prevention of diabetic foot wounds. Foot & Ankle International. 2005;**26**(1):5-14

[41] Laborde JM. Tendon lengthening for neuropathic foot problems. Orthopedics. 2010;**33**(5):319-326. DOI: 10.3928/01477447-20100329-26

[42] Hsu JD, Hsu CL. In: Jahss MH, editor. Disorders of the Foot. Philadelphia, PA: WB Saunders; 1982

[43] Stromeyer L. In: Rang M, editor. Anthology of Orthopaedics. Edinburgh, Scotland: Livingstone, Ltd.; 1996. pp. 212-215

[44] Vulpius O, Stoffel A. Orthopaedische Operationslehre. 2nd ed. Stuttgart: Ferdinand Enke; 1920

[45] Mayerson M, Papa J, Eaton K, Wilson K. The total-contact cast for management of neuropathic plantar ulceration of the foot. JBJS. 1992;**74**:261-269

[46] Poala JD, Faglia E, Caminiti M, Clerici G, Ninkovic S, Deanesi V. Ulcer recurrence following first ray amputation in diabetic patients. Diabetes Care. 2003;**26**(6):1874-1878

[47] Krause FG, deVries G, Meakin C, Kalla TP, Younger ASE. Outcome of transmetatarsal amputation in diabetics using antibiotic beads. Foot & Ankle International. 2009;**6**:4486-4483

[48] Pinzur M, Kaminsky M, Sage R, Cronin R, Osterman H. Amputation at the middle of the foot. JBJS. 1986;**68**(7):1061-1064

[49] Lieberman JR, Jacobs RL, Goldstock L, Durham J, Fuchs MD. Chopart amputation with percutaneous heel cord lengthening. Clinical Orthopaedics and Related Research. 1993;**296**(Nov.):86-91

[50] Hirsch AT, Haskal ZJ, Hertzer NR, et al. ACC/AHA 2005 practice guidelines for the management of patients with peripheral arterial disease. Circulation. 2006;**113**(11):e463-e654

[51] Hoppe DJ, Schemitsch ED, Morshed S, Tornetta P, Bhandari M. Hierarchy of evidence: Where observational studies fit in and why we need them. JBJS. 2009;**91**(53):2-9

[52] Lountzis N, Parenti J, Cush G, Urick M, Miller F. Percutaneuos flexor

tenotomy office procedure for diabetic toe ulcerations. Wounds. 2007;**19**(3):64-68

[53] Johnson JE. Operative treatment of neuropathic arthropathy of the foot and ankle. JBJS. 1998;**80**(11):1700-1709

[54] Meyerson MS, Henderson MR, Sarby T, Short KW. Management of midfoot diabetic neuropathy. Foot & Ankle International. 1994;**15**(5):233-241

[55] Thomas JL, Huffman L. Charcot foot deformity: Surgical treatment options. Wounds. Malvern, PA: Global Learning Network; 2008. Available from: www.woundresearch.com/article/8476

[56] Fabrin J, Larsen K, Holstein PE. Long-term follow-up in diabetic Charcot feet with spontaneous onset. Diabetes Care. 2000;**23**(6):796-800

[57] Laborde JM, Philbin TM, Chandler PJ, Daigre J. Preliminary results of primary gastrocnemius-soleus recession for midfoot Charcot arthropathy. Foot and Ankle Specialist. 2016;**9**(2):140-144. DOI: 10.1177/1938640015607051

[58] van Netten JJ, Price PE, Lavery LA, Mnteiro-Soares M, Rasmussen A, Jubiz Y, et al. The international working group on the diabetic foot. Prevention of foot ulcers in the at-risk patient with diabetes: A systematic review. Diabetes/Metabolism Research and Reviews. 2016;**32**(Suppl. 1):84-98

[59] Rush SM, Ford LA, Hamilton GA. Morbidity associated with high gastrocnemius recession. The Journal of Foot and Ankle Surgery. 2006;**45**(3):156-160

[60] Myers TG, Lowery NJ, Frykberg WDK. Ankle and hindfoot fusions: Comparison of outcomes in patients with and without diabetes. Foot & Ankle International. 2012;**33**(1):20-28

[61] Belatti DA, Phisitkul P. Declines in lower extremity amputation in the Medicare population, 2000-2010. Foot & Ankle International. 2013;**34**(7):923-931. DOI: 101177/1071100713475357

[62] Cychoz CC, Phisitkul P, Belatti DA, Wukich DK. Preventative and therapeutic strategies for diabetic foot ulcers. Foot & Ankle International. 2016;**37**(3):334-343. DOI: 10.1177/1071100715611951

[63] Tiruveedhula M, Graham A, Thapar A, Dindayal S, Mulcahay M. Outcomes of Tendo-Achilles lengthening and weight-bearing total contact cast for management of early midfoot Charcot neuropathy. Journal of Clinical Orthopaedics and Trauma. 2021;**17**:128-138

[64] Yammine K, Assi C. Conservative surgical options for the treatment of forefoot diabetic ulcers: An evidence based review. JBJS Reviews. 2020;**8**(6):e0162. DOI: 10.2106/JBJS.RVW.19.00162

[65] Yammine K, Assi C. Surgery vs. nonsurgical methods in treating neuropathic plantar forefoot ulcers: A meta-analysis. The International Journal of Lower Extremity Wounds. 2020;**21**(1):7-17. DOI: 10.1177/1534734620923425

[66] Bowers AL, Castro MD. The mechanics behind the image: Foot and ankle pathology associated with gastrocnemius contracture. Seminars in Musculoskeletal Radiology. 2007;**11**(1):83-90

[67] Van Gils CC, Roeder B. The effect of ankle equinus upon the diabetic

foot. Clinics in Podiatric Medicine and Surgery. 2002;**19**(3):391-409

[68] Anderson JG, Bohay DR, Eller EB, Witt BL. Gastrocnemius recession. Foot and Ankle Clinics. 2014;**19940**:767-786. DOI: 10.1016/j.fcl.2014.09.001

[69] Kirane YM, Michelson JD, Sharkey NA. Contribution of the flexor hallicis longus to loading of the first metatarsal and the first metatarsophalangeal joint. Foot & Ankle International. 2008;**29**(4):367-377

[70] de Prado M, Ripolli PL, Golano P. Minmally invasive foot surgery. About Your Health Publishers; 2009. pp. 61-255. ISBN-13:978-84-613-1609-0

[71] Holme TJ, Sivaloganathan SS, Patel B, Kunasingam K. Third generation minimally invasive Chevron akin for hallux valgus. Foot & Ankle International. 2020;**41**(1):50-56

Chapter 5

Mitigating Diabetic Foot Ulcers: The Effect of Diet and Microbiome

Steven Coon

Abstract

To truly eliminate the possibility of diabetic foot ulcers, the elimination of the symptoms of diabetes is essential. There are many forms of diabetes and there is no one diet that is effective for all patients. It is essential that a proper diet is utilized and for most diabetic patients a reduction in weight and the restoration of a properly balanced microbiota can eliminate the devastating effects of diabetes including foot ulcers. This review examines in detail the different types of diets, and how they affect the host and the microbiota to eliminate as much as possible the risk of foot ulcers. Microbiota, diet, incretins, and insulin all directly affect the deposition of fats which causes insulin insensitivity and diabetes in most patients.

Keywords: incretin, SCFA, diabetes, carbohydrates, fats

1. Introduction

Type 2 Diabetes Mellites (TTDM), which is approximately 95% of all diabetic patients in 2010, affected 280 million (approximately 6.2%) of the world's population and is thought to increase to 7.5% by 2030 [1, 2]. This is thought to be due to an increase in the number of obese individuals which leads primarily to an increase in their incidence of TTDM. Most scientists and medical professionals believe that obesity begins at a BMI of 30 and severe obesity at a BMI of 40 but many studies are now suggesting that BMI is not a truly accurate measure of obesity [3]. Most TTDM patients are obese and about 2-3 percent of patients have current active foot ulcers and up to 25% will eventually develop foot ulcers [4]. This occurs as a result of uncontrolled diabetes that interferes with wound healing, reduces pain response, and causes problems with proper blood circulation. Although ulcers can actually occur anywhere on the body, the feet are most vulnerable.

The chief cause of foot ulcerations is due to diabetic neuropathy. High blood glucose levels cause arteries to harden and develop plaques that limit blood flow to tissues including nerves and the heart. This causes reduced nutrient and oxygen uptake by the nerves causing neuropathy. Diabetic neuropathy affects both the somatic as well as autonomic nervous systems resulting in a complex group of pathophysiological disorders. One of the manifestations of these disorders in the diabetic foot which can result in anatomical and physiological changes in the foot such as ulcerations and infections because of a lack of wound healing and a delayed immune response. Since the feet are frequently covered and the soles are exposed to compression from walking feet when it comes to ulcerations, the feet are the most vulnerable part of the body. Wound healing is slowed for several reasons. Hyperglycemia is a contributing factor to atherosclerosis. This limits the blood flow, especially to the heart but also to any wounds and the feet tend to be even more susceptible [5, 6]. Nerve damage can cause a loss of sensation in the foot and peripheral vascular disease that can go unnoticed. If these conditions become severe enough, this can cause further damage to bone, joints, and soft tissue and if not treated can eventually lead to amputation [7, 8]. Life expectancy following amputation is about 50% within five years [9, 10] although many of those deaths could be due to contributing comorbidities related to diabetes-induced cardiovascular disease [3].

It would seem to suggest that control of diabetes and its symptoms would be the best way to prevent ulcerations. However, it does not fully eliminate the risk [11]. There are two major forms - Type 1 and Type 2 diabetes but there are other less well-known forms as well which include gestational and atypical diabetes. They have very similar symptoms, but their causes can be quite different and are often misdiagnosed [12]. If the weight and diet are left unchanged despite control of diabetic symptoms, there is still a risk of ulcerations, especially on the feet. To eliminate the risk altogether, the weight must be lost, and diabetes must go away completely to eliminate the risks.

One can certainly do regular foot inspections to avoid the worse complications of foot ulcers and be sure that their diabetes is under control. Metformin is the most used drug to treat diabetic patients but other drugs such as incretin agonists particularly GLP-1 and DPP4 inhibitors are also being used and often in combination with Metformin [13].

Some patients also use insulin injections as well. None of these drugs ensure that diabetes can be controlled at all times which makes foot inspections required.

Children can also develop foot ulcers and more and more studies are showing that the mother can contribute to these problems [14]. Cesarean sections rather than vaginal births can alter the seeding of microbiota during the birth process. In addition, the mother if she is diabetic or has elevated blood sugar, these sugars can be passed along to the infant during breastfeeding causing the infant to have elevated blood sugars [14]. Studies have been performed up to about four months of age which is the median age at which infants begin to eat solid food. Infants were divided into four groups based on cesarean versus vaginal birth and breast milk versus formula and found that vaginal births with breast milk fared better when their microbiota were compared [15]. Breast milk also contains a great number of good bacteria as well from the skin microbiota that can be missing if the mother fails to breastfeed [14]. These combinations can lead to obesity and diabetes in young children and eventually to the complications of diabetes previously described for adults including foot ulcers.

2. Incretins and diabetes

Incretins such as GLP1 and GIP are released during a meal. When one overeats, there is number of effects. Glucose and other nutrients stimulate incretin release when they are absorbed which continues to stimulate even more absorption. The nutrients are absorbed regardless of whether they are necessary for bodily functions and much of it is directed into glycolysis to eventually produce ATP, shuttled into glycogen, or stimulated by incretins to be digested and absorbed into adipocytes and stored as fat (see **Figure 1**).

Incretins also stimulate the release of insulin as well and as incretin levels rise because of overeating, insulin levels rise as well. GLP-1 is released from L-cells of the small intestine [16]. One of the effects of increased secretion of insulin however can cause insulin receptors to desensitize and become nonresponsive and promoting insulin resistance. This leads to high blood glucose levels leading to diabetes. Increased amounts of insulin, incretin agonists, DTT inhibitors, and other drugs are

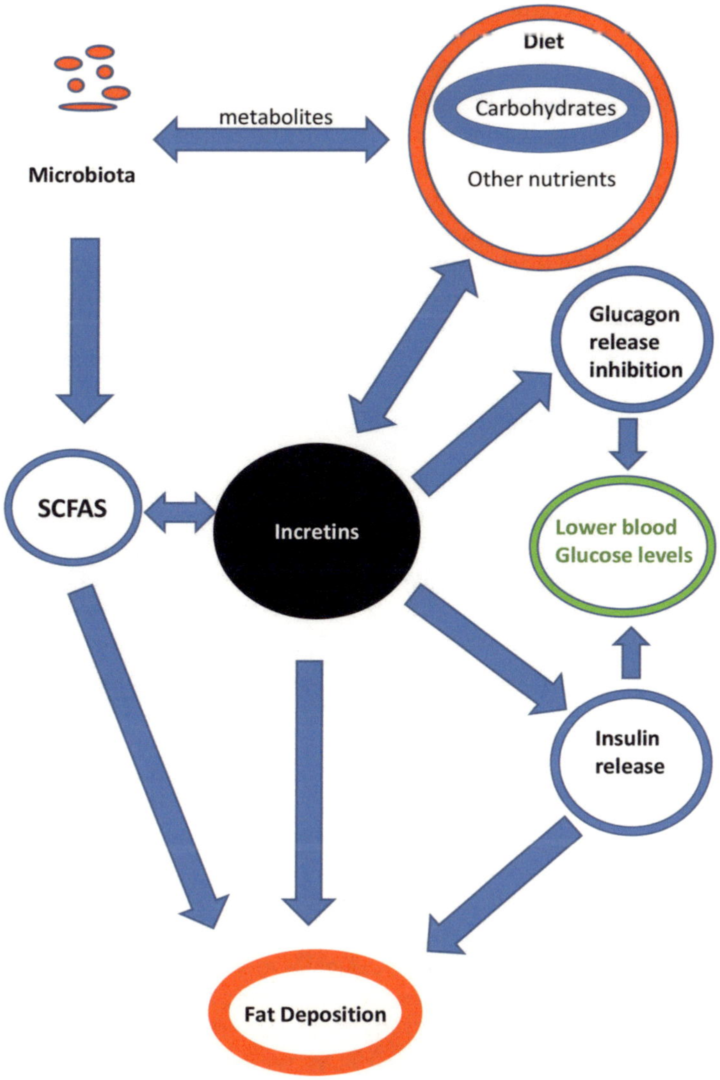

Figure 1.
Represented above is a simplified diagram of blood glycemic control and fat deposition. Incretins are at the heart of control and not just involved in stimulating insulin release. Incretins can have direct effects on fat deposition. In the energy balance mode and carbohydrate – insulin model of obesity it appears the influence of diet and SCFAs are not emphasized enough on the impact of glycemic control and fat deposition. Microbiota and the production of SCFAs have a profound effect on insulin release. Although carbohydrates have a large effect on secretion of insulin, other nutrients also have an effect. Although insulin can stimulate the production fat in adipocytes, incretins and SCFAs can have a direct effect as well.

designed to increase the amounts of insulin without fixing the underlying physiological causes. For TTDM and similar forms of diabetes, this is possible but for TT1 this is more difficult and in most cases impossible. So, depending on the cause, the diets and effects of microbiota are quite different.

GLP-1 and GIP both stimulate the secretion of insulin from the Beta cells of the Pancreas, yet they have different effects on obesity and fat deposition and different studies are making the functions unclear [17]. GLP-1 directly inhibits appetite and food intake and GLP-1 antagonists have been developed into drugs that can help glycemic control. GIP however lacks these functions and although some studies have used agonists to reduce weight gain, also antagonists have shown the same effect [17–20]. In addition, GIP receptor knockout mice fail to gain weight even when fed a high-fat diet [21]. GIP is released when glucose and proteins are absorbed which then promote additional absorption [22, 23].

Incretin control is what causes insulin release and increased amounts can lead to diabetes and eventually the complications that eventually lead to foot ulcers. Rises in incretins particularly GIP can contribute to weight gain by increasing absorption of nutrients and fat deposition (**Figure 1**). Control of incretin release could modulate and maintain controlled diabetes and less of a risk of ulcers. Even before one eats a meal, incretins such as GLP-1 and GIP are released in anticipation of glucose absorption. But the evidence is rather ambiguous [24]. Some studies show that even the sweet taste of food (even if it's an artificial sweetener) can trigger incretin release during the cephalic phase of digestion [1, 25]. Others have shown no release of insulin during the cephalic phase [26, 27].

3. The effects of diet on diabetic foot ulcers

There are two prevailing and compelling theories of obesity and diabetes, but they are somewhat opposing theories neither of which explains entirely the complexity of obesity and glycemic control [28, 29]. The first is called the energy balance model (EBM) and the carbohydrate-insulin model (CIM). Although most scientists may be in favor of the EBM, the recent studies on the CIM and the effect and results of a low carbohydrate diet are compelling. Depending on the strategy of each model, determines the diet that would work best. Diets can influence incretin release and provide the proper amounts of SCFAs (see **Figure 1**).

Less than 10% of all diabetic patients have type I diabetes or similar atypical diabetic diseases. Type I diabetic patients should already be on a special diet to help control their blood glucose levels. One should monitor the intake of carbohydrates and concentrate on low glycemic foods and beverages. One should be aware that sugar-free foods and beverages do not necessarily mean carbohydrate free. Patients that fall into this category have diabetes because their pancreas beta cells do not produce sufficient amounts of insulin [30] to regulate their blood glucose levels. But there is no one meal plan that fits all. For TTDM patients, insulin insensitivity is the problem, and to relieve those symptoms usually a reduction in weight is necessary. This means a reduction in calorie intake, especially of dense energy foods such as fatty foods, and perhaps even lifestyle change.

Diabetes diets are certainly important and those that have diabetic symptoms should follow these guidelines. A carbohydrate-reduced diet is recommended but carbohydrates are found in many foods with grains such as bread, pasta, milk, any sweets that contain processed sugars, fruit, and even some vegetables that are high in starches (white and sweet potatoes, corn, peas, squash, and turnips). However, many of these foods contain many necessary nutrients and cannot necessarily be completely excluded. Most vegetables including potatoes contain vital amounts of fiber that essential bacteria that are part of the microbiota require.

Fiber is also an essential part of the diet and consists of starches that are non-digestible or less digestible than other forms of carbohydrates. In humans, cellulose and chitin are not digested like they are in ruminants such as cattle or other multi-stomach animals that consume grass or other plants. In humans, amylose even though it is a straight chain of glucose residues, and its secondary structure makes it more difficult to digest those other forms such as amylopectin that is found in plants and glycogen that is found in animals. Therefore, amylose is often considered a resistant starch, and foods that contain more amylose, and less amylopectin are considered low glycemic and will not cause glucose levels to rise as quickly or as much and can be a benefit for diabetic patients [31, 32]. Potatoes are already being developed to contain a higher amylose/amylopectin ratio by hybridizing with other strains while at the same time increasing their protein and amino acid content [31]. Not all of these new plants are commercially available as yet and potatoes such as huckleberry gold although available are more expensive than the more common commercially available varieties. Although these potatoes have been reported to have higher amylose/amylopectin ratios, it still remains to be seen if the cooking methods will have an effect and if the varieties will taste good enough to be accepted as substitutes. Until then, the recommended foods include Grains, beans (canned baked beans tend to have sugars added), rice, pasta, and starchy vegetables are actually recommended because of their high fiber content even though they may not be low glycemic.

In addition, it is rapidly becoming more important to consume vegetables because of their high polyphenol content as well. Polyphenols are a large group of plant metabolites that have many medicinal properties including antidiabetic effects. Polyphenols have been shown to decrease blood glucose levels and increase insulin secretion and sensitivity [33, 34].

The release of digested carbohydrates releases glucose that is absorbed which can raise blood glucose levels. Proteins and fats have not been found to affect diabetic patients, but any weight gain can contribute to diabetes and insulin resistance. Type one diabetes does not typically cause insulin resistance, but some type one diabetic patients have become overweight, and more than a third now have an increased risk of chronic kidney disease [35]. It has been shown that the increased blood glucose levels damage the delicate blood vessels, and many develop high blood pressure as well which can damage the vessels as well [30], which could contribute to insulin resistance. Since there is no one diet fits all, the current diet for a particular individual depends on age, weight, and the activity of the individual. It is suggested that a registered dietician may be the best way to design a diet. Typically, an individual should not consume more than 2000 calories per day, and no more than half should be from carbohydrates. Typically, also one gram of carbohydrates has about 4 calories, but these are only estimates. There are general guidelines for patients with diabetes. Watching portion size and calories are recommended for any diabetes diet. Reducing the intake of fried foods, sweets, salts and fats is a part of any diabetes diet. In some cases, even eating less more often can stabilize your glucose levels in the blood. One thing however to keep in mind is that not all calories are the same. Calories coming from energy-dense diets will predispose individuals to weight gain irrespective of the nutrient content of the food consumed [36, 37].

3.1 The ketogenic diet

The most popular of diabetes-related diets are the ketogenic diet. Ketogenic diets are frequently higher fat, lower fiber diets that have lower carbohydrates making it easier to control diabetes and induce weight loss [37–39]. Low fiber diets, however, will not restore normal microbiota which contributes to obesity therefore it is not a long-term solution that should be discontinued once the normal weight is achieved. There are different forms of these diets but essentially even less carbohydrate is consumed in favor of additional protein. This is known as nutritional ketosis which is a normal biological process that may in fact reduce weight and eventually be beneficial to the individual [37, 38]. But it would only be normal when the diabetes is under control and blood glucose levels are normal. However, this is different than ketoacidosis which can occur in diabetic patients where the diabetes is not under control when insulin levels are too low, and glucose cannot be absorbed into cells instead the body uses fats for fuel. In this case, there is a sharp unhealthy rise in ketones in the blood which in turn causes the blood to become more acidic [38]. This condition can be fatal if not treated. Keto diets as well can lead to nutrient deficiencies in calcium, magnesium, vitamin D, and folic acid. The vast majority of TTDM patients are obese and only when their obesity is also under control and reduced will their diabetes symptoms disappear [37, 38]. Nevertheless, long-term use of the ketogenic diet has not been well studied and can have serious side effects. It has been shown that this diet while preventing some cancers can cause renal cancer and tumor growth in integument and other epithelial tissues [38, 40]. Ketogenic diets are often high in fat and low in fiber. That kind of diet will cause LDL levels to rise to lead to serious heart and cardiovascular diseases such as atherosclerosis. If the fats are reduced in favor of higher protein levels that can lead to serious kidney diseases and kidney stones [37].

Type one diabetes and TTDM patients can both benefit from a ketogenic diet, but the endpoints will be different. For TTDM patients, a ketogenic diet could restore normal weight and therefore usually relieve the symptoms of diabetes. For type one, the risk of ketoacidosis is significantly higher and so needs more careful monitoring. The Ketogenic diet can benefit diabetic patients because it reduces the glucose levels in the blood, lowers blood pressure, and can contribute to weight loss [37, 39].

4. Other diets

4.1 The low-carb diet

A low-carb diet is different than the ketogenic diet because it is less limiting in the amount of carbohydrates. You don't have to give up carbohydrates because you have diabetes. Atkins or South Beach are low-carb diets that are easier to comply with, and many patients still benefit from them. Studies show that this diet could be the first step in managing the disease [41].

4.2 Mediterranean diet

This diet promotes fruits and vegetables as well as fish, chicken, nuts, olive oil, legumes, and whole grains with a reduction of red meat, butter, and salt. Studies have shown that diet can help keep blood sugar levels under control. You can have some alcohol with meals as well [42].

DOI: http://dx.doi.org/10.5772/intechopen.106629

4.3 Dash diet

Dieticians recommend this eating plan usually as a way to control hypertension. The diet consists of fruits, vegetables, low-fat dairy, whole grains, lean meats, fish, nuts, and beans. (It does allow for some sweets in moderation.) Studies have found that it can improve insulin sensitivity when it is part of an overall weight loss program with exercise [43].

4.4 Zone diet

Meals are designed to contain 40% carbs, 30% protein, and 30% fat. Carbs are ranked as good or bad based on the glycemic index. Foods like chicken and barley are recommended but not potatoes and egg yolks. Studies have found it had a positive effect on glycemic control and waist size, so it may be a good choice. Ask your doctor about it (zonediet.com).

4.5 Paleo diet

The idea behind this diet is to eat the way early humans did before modern farming. The diet consists of no dairy, refined sugar, grains, or legumes, and no processed vegetable oils like soybean oil or canola oil. You can have fruits and vegetables, lean meats (preferably grass-fed), fish, nuts, and seeds. Using this, diet studies show this eating strategy can improve blood sugar and diabetes (thepaleodiet.com [44]).

4.6 Vegetarian/vegan

Limiting or avoiding animal products like chicken, fish, and yogurt may be a healthier way to live for some individuals. However serious deficiencies in nutrients can occur. The diet generally restricts meat and poultry but in some cases, dairy, eggs, or fish are allowed to prevent these deficiencies (Mayo Clinic; Vegetarian Diet: How to get the best nutrition). Research shows that people who eat a plant-based diet get more fiber and take in fewer calories and fat than nonvegetarians. This would bring diabetes under control and restore the normal microbiota balance however deficiencies in Vitamin B12, Omega 3 fatty acids, iron, zinc, and iodine can develop if the diet is not properly monitored.

5. Microbiota

The large intestine (colon) is populated by a large number of bacterial, archaeal, protozoan, viral and fungal species that are collectively known as the gut microbiota. The number of species ranges from hundreds to tens of thousands that outnumber the human genome by at least 100:1 and are known as the second human genome. The microbiota, especially the bacterial species, forms a community of organisms that metabolize nondigestible carbohydrates, plant cell wall material, and other oligosaccharides that make up dietary fiber, and they produce a wide variety of metabolites including short-chain fatty acids (SCFAs) [45]. Other substances, especially the polyphenols in the diet, serve as substrates for the microbiota. Other secondary molecules include vitamins, cholesterol, and their derivatives, along with the other remaining cell wall components such as lipopolysaccharides, which can also be found as metabolites formed by the microbiota [46]. A high fat, low fiber diet reduces SCFAs producing increasing the numbers *Firmicutes* and decreasing the numbers of the *Bacteroidetes* phyla, and also decreasing the level of SCFAs (since there is less fiber) and the synthesis of other essential metabolites [47]. SCFAs such as acetate, propionate, and butyrate are synthesized as byproducts of resistance starch metabolism by the microbiota. On the other hand, these bacteria can also metabolize histidine into imidazole propionate which actually can modulate host inflammation, metabolism and cause insulin resistance [48].

To a certain extent, antibiotics, certain diseases (e.g., inflammatory bowel diseases; IBD), and the genetics of the host may contribute to dysbiosis; however, an individual's diet has a major impact on the growth and maturation of the microbiota [49]. SCFAs have distinct effects on colon epithelia, specific transport and signaling mechanisms, and profound effects on a human's health including diabetes.

5.1 The chemistry and metabolism of SCFAs

SCFAs are mostly aliphatic carboxylic acids that have a carbon chain of six or less. A few SCFAs are branched and synthesized from various amino acids but contribute only about 5% of the overall SCFAs produced.

The microbiota consists mainly of *Bacteroidetes* and *Firmicutes* (combined are approximately 90% of the gut microbiota), while the remaining bacteria consist of Actinobacteria, Proteobacteria, and *Verrucomicrobiota*. Amazingly, even within the first month of life, the gastrointestinal (GI) tracts of children are colonized by different species of *Bacteroidetes* and *Firmicutes* at a much lower level. A child's GI tract begins germ-free but accumulates additional numbers of species until the child achieves adulthood. Diet, geographic location, and the genetics of the individual are all contributors to the microbiota colonization of the adult GI tract. In addition, it is now hypothesized that microbiota present in the birth canal during childbirth contributes to gastrointestinal colonization and those children born through the Cesarian section have more health problems than those who do not. Breastfeeding rather than simple formula (not exactly the same diet) also modulates the microbial species that colonize the GI tracts since breastmilk has bacteria from the skin microbiota. Therefore, it is conceivable that the diet can have a profound influence on the child's microbiota population and health. It is even more conceivable that an increase in childhood obesity could be influenced by changes and/or deficits in the developing microbiota [49–51].

Nondigested carbohydrates that are used as nutrients by the microbiota of the GI tract are referred to as prebiotics [52]. Enteric nutrition is given to certain patients as a supplement during their hospital stay to prevent malnutrition. Such treatments frequently result in diarrhea. Once prebiotics are added to the enteric nutrition, the symptoms of diarrhea disappear [53]. Thus, a diet with a proper prebiotic level is critical for maintaining a proper *Firmicutes* to *Bacteroidetes* ratio. Conversely, a high fat, low fiber (i.e., low prebiotic) diet will increase the *Firmicutes* to *Bacteroidetes* ratio [49]. It is well known that SCFAs are produced by the microbiota and when they are absorbed, the SCFAs stimulate $Na+$/water absorption [54]. Therefore, prebiotics are essential to maintain a proper ratio for any diet. Prebiotics are those foods that contain different types of nondigestible fiber as a fuel source for microbiota. The prebiotics include mostly vegetables such as artichokes, leeks, garlic, onions, asparagus, wheat bran/flour, bananas, and chicory root. It is important to note that when vegetables are cooked they lose at least a third of their fiber content [52].

Once SCFAs are produced, most are transported into colonocytes and are metabolized by the colonocytes as a nutrient for cell growth and metabolism. Very little of the SCFAs are transported into the systemic circulation. Acetate levels are likely high enough to have effects on the other organs, but very little if any, butyrate or propionate is thought to leave the portal blood and liver [55]. A limited amount is produced and absorbed in the small intestine, but the colon is certainly the major source [56]. Receptors for SCFAs exist in most of the major organs including the gastrointestinal tract. In the intestine and colon, SCFAs are linked to motility and maintenance of the epithelial barrier. SCFAs stimulate water absorption, while at the same time increasing motility, maintaining the epithelial barrier and therefore preventing constipation and diarrhea [57]. When entering into the systemic circulation, SCFAs also have profound effects on whole body health and metabolism. SCFAs are the source of fuel for the heart and the cardiovascular system, they control body weight and insulin release, and are precursors for lipid and glucose production in the liver (gluconeogenesis). Commensal bacteria have a number of health benefits which include the development of the gastrointestinal tract and other tissues such as the central nervous system, maintaining the immune system, and increasing metabolism [58]. Therefore, an imbalance or dysregulation of microbiota populations could disrupt normal metabolism and water balance and result in obesity, diabetes, and its symptoms and complications such as foot ulcers.

The major SCFAs produced are acetate (C2), propionate (C3), and butyrate (C4) which contain two, three, and four carbons, respectively. These SCFAs are mainly synthesized by the Firmicutes species *Lactobacillus* and also the *Actinomycetota* species *Bifidobacteria*. *Bacteroidetes* bacteria can also produce SCFAs but at lower levels. The SCFAs act as the primary source of energy for colonocytes. Different species of bacteria with different metabolic steps are responsible for the formation of each of the SCFAs. None of the bacteria have all of the necessary enzymes to produce all three of the SCFAs directly from dietary fiber. Nondigestible carbohydrates enter the citric acid cycle of bacteria at different points in different bacteria. Propionate is formed from succinyl-CoA, an intermediate of the citric acid cycle, as well as lactate and propanediol. Acetate and butyrate are formed from acetyl-CoA [59, 60]. In addition to entering the citric acid cycle and being used as an energy source, SCFAs also have profound epigenetic effects to increase the rate of gene transcription by inhibiting histone deacetylase (HDAC) activity [61]. The SCFAs affect many genes that regulate transcription and colonocyte homeostasis [62, 63]. These accumulated epigenetic events are thought to increase the incidence of colorectal cancer [64, 65]. Butyrate is synthesized from acetate, while propionate is synthesized by butyrate-producing bacterial species such as *Faecalibacterium, Eubacterium, and Anaerostipes* [66, 67]. Additionally, to absorption (i.e., about 95% of SCFAs produced), some of the SCFAs are excreted in the feces [60]. The amount of SCFAs produced can vary greatly by the content and type of dietary fiber, and the number and species of bacteria. Other factors such as antibiotics, bypass surgery, and stress can also alter the microbiota species composition and SCFAs production. Local sanitation and the introduction of microbes into the diet determine whether the proper microbiota is developed in the GI tract. Amazingly, people in countries with the best sanitation introduce fewer microbes into the microbiota, which consequently leads to dysbiosis and diseases such as obesity and diabetes [49].

SCFAs can exert physiological function either during transport across the colonocytes or by binding to their receptors located on the gastrointestinal mucosa. A number of orphan G-protein-linked receptors were discovered and initially had no known ligands [68]. However, later studies demonstrated that SCFAs activated several of these G-protein-linked receptors, and several of them are identified to present in the mucosa of intestine and colon [69]. They include the G-protein coupled receptor (GPR) GPR43 (acetate and propionate) and GPR41 (propionate and butyrate), which have about 40% homology across species [70]. GPR43 and GPR41 are also known as free fatty acid receptors, (FFAR) FFAR2, and FFAR3, respectively. Acetate and propionate are ligands for GPR43 (FFAR2), while propionate and butyrate are ligands for GPR42 (FFAR3) [45]. Butyrate also binds to GPR109a, which is distributed along the colon, T-cells, and the microglia. GPR43 is highly expressed in immune cells, adipose tissue (stimulates fat deposition), distal ileum (increases motility, and stimulates peptide-YY (PYY) and glucagon-like peptide-1 (GLP-1) secretion), skeletal muscle, and the heart [71] that are tissues all involved in diabetes and obesity. Therefore, during dysbiosis and diabetes when there is a lack of SCFAs this could contribute to a decrease in immune responses and cause cardiovascular disorders. The main function of GPR43 is to maintain energy homeostasis within the body, GPR43 increases energy released by improving glucose tolerance and increasing energy utilization within the body [72]. GPR43 is also present in pancreatic β-cells and stimulates insulin secretion, which in turn increases glucose absorption into the tissues to aid increased energy utilization. These aspects were demonstrated using GPR43 knockout mice [73, 74]. Therefore, when SCFAs are not synthesized j in sufficient quantities then that would result in difficulties in maintaining normal energy homeostasis and glucose utilization. Although most of the SCFAs are utilized in the colon, more dietary fiber consumption, resulting in greater amounts of SCFAs, gets absorbed into the systemic circulation and thus interacts with other tissue receptors. Although further studies are required, it is likely that SCFAs increase body metabolism, as high fiber diets result in weight loss and reduce blood lipid levels. Additionally, increases in HDL levels are observed, which lowers the chances of atherosclerosis, but an increase in blood cholesterol levels has been shown in some studies [47, 75–77]. However, this reported evidence indicates that SCFAs activate receptors that release GLP-1 and increase insulin secretion to regulate blood glucose levels [70]. In the pulmonary system, SCFAs protect against inflammation by activating the GPR41 and reducing hematopoiesis and infiltration of immune cells [78]. Loss of these functions would result in weight gain, cardiovascular disorders, and insulin resistance.

Altered microbiota populations have been detected in several diseases including obesity and conditions resulting from the overuse of antibiotics. The overuse of antibiotics has been shown to decrease Bacteroidetes and increase Firmicutes [14]. Metabolic activity of Bacteroidetes and Firmicutes taxa determined by 16s RNA analyses revealed that the Firmicutes tend to be more active than that of Bacteroidetes taxa. Even with the cessation of antibiotic treatment, some species, mainly Firmicutes, never return to normal levels [76, 79].

When microbiota utilize fats and metabolize less fiber in the diet, the microbiota synthesize fewer SCFAs but also produce metabolites that contribute to obesity. When the ratio of *Firmicutes* to *Bacteroidetes* increases that contributes to an increased risk of diabetes and obesity [80]. However, a change in the ratio does not always lead to diabetes [81, 82] because there can be regional differences in the expression of the microbiota in lean and obese individuals which likely depends on the diet at that locale [83, 84]. However, dietary requirements for modulation of diabetes may not have enough impact but it is certainly important since increases in fiber in the diet reduced the symptoms of diabetes in patients [80, 85]. Many of these food items rich in fiber also contain large amounts of sugars and carbohydrates. It is interesting that with weight loss comes changes in microbiota, but the research design many times do not reflect enough which came first, the change in weight or the change in microbiota making interpretation of results difficult.

There are two major phyla of bacteria that are present in the gut microbiome. The ratio of these bacteria is balanced in healthy lean individuals. Firmicutes are considered to be the "bad" bacteria but they are the major phyla that produce the short chain fatty acids needed as a fuel source for the colon [86, 87]. Without the SCFA when the Bacteroidetes become the dominant phyla with fewer *Firmicutes* colon will become more permeable to bacterial infections and diseases such as Inflammatory Bowel Disease although some report even *Bacteroidetes* are also reduced [88]. Other phyla include Actinobacteria as they increase significantly decrease the risk of developing diabetes [89], *Proteobacteria* increases have been linked to dysbiosis and may not cause diabetes but those with diabetes have increased amounts, particularly in TTDM [90], and *Verrucomicrobia* is also increased in diabetic patients [91].

High fat low fiber diets tend to diminish and cause dysbiosis of the colon microbiota. Fermented foods are considered to be among the best foods that can replace or restore the normal balance of microbiota in humans [14]. Yogurt is considered to be among the best, but only recently have there been any definitive studies. *Bifidobacterium animalis* and *Lactobacillus* species are said to be the most beneficial and are found in yogurt and other fermented milk products [14, 92]; however, immune deficient patients should avoid yogurts and other fermented milk products since they could be susceptible to a fatal form of septicemia [93]. These short-chain fatty acids (SCFAs) are not just linked as a fuel source for colonocytes in the large intestine but also to proper immune responses and proper intestinal permeability to prevent bacterial infections [88]. Parasitic infections which can result from increased permeability such as toxoplasmosis, hydatidosis, and cysticercosis infect a large population worldwide. *Toxoplasma gondii* in the pancreas could damage the pancreatic cells. Hence, insulin secretion would be affected which leads to an increased risk of diabetes [94].

6. Other microbiomes

The gut microbiome is by far the most important when it comes to diabetes and obesity, but it is becoming clear that other microbiomes may have effects as well. Small intestinal bacterial overgrowth syndrome (SIBO), *Heliobacter pylori*, and the oral microbiome are now thought to contribute as well. SIBO and H. pylori are often comorbidities for diabetic patients.

SIBO is an upset of the natural balance of microbiota in the small intestine. It can be the result of enteric nervous system disorders such as IBS and because of nausea and abdominal pain usually result in weight loss, loss of appetite, bloating and diarrhea, and malnutrition. SIBO causes increased blood glucose levels and insulin resistance and worsening glycemic control [95]. Other investigators though believe that it is diabetes that causes SIBO. About a third of diabetic patients also have SIBO. [96] and is diagnosed by a simple hydrogen breath test. However, unless the SIBO can be controlled, these patients will have greater difficulty in controlling their diabetes and will have a higher risk of foot ulcers [96].

Heliobacter pylori infections in the stomach also increase the likelihood of TTDM. Causal contact and contaminated food or water can transmit the disease. It is believed that the infections cause the release of gastric hormones and gastrointestinal inflammation that leads eventually to insulin resistance and diabetes [97].

Oral microbiomes are now being examined and studies show that this microbiome is also involved in the progression of diabetes and obesity. *Actinobacteria* levels are seriously depressed in diabetic patients and *Firmicute/Bacteroidetes* ratios have increased just as in gut microbiota in TTDM patients [89, 98, 99].

7. Host genetics

Genetics can affect many areas of human physiology that can affect the progression of diabetic foot ulcers. There are genes that can affect not just obesity but also diabetes. As many as 20 different genes have been associated with type I diabetes [100]. It is usually an autoimmune disease passed on from parents to offspring. However, there is a greater chance of parents having children who also have Type 1 Diabetes however there is no evidence that it's not simply due to similar diets and living conditions since they are likely to live all in the same place. For type two diabetic patients the atypical types have been directly linked to mutations in certain genes but that only accounts for a small percentage of diabetic patients. MODY type diabetes is all the result of a single mutation causing a lack of glycemic control [12]. Nevertheless, some investigators believe that genes only predispose an individual to obesity and do not guarantee the condition and that environment plays just as important a role in diabetes/obesity phenotype. Now, there is also evidence that *Firmicute* family *Christensenellaceae* increased in numbers in lean non-diabetic individuals and is directly associated with the host genome [101]. It was demonstrated that in identical twins, the microbiota was more similar than twins that were not identical [102] which suggests genetics has an important role in determining correct balance of microbiota and therefore maintenance of energy balance, proper weight, and glycemic control.

8. Conclusion

Diabetic foot ulcers have protocols for treatment and prevention but ultimately the only way to prevent them entirely is to address the diabetes of the patients involved. Although this review is not entirely a comprehensive review of diabetes, it is clear that its prevention is not a simple matter especially if its cause and treatment are not necessarily well defined. Since there are two prevailing theories of its cause and there are different types of diabetes and diets the effects of microbiota and diet are not going to be the same for everyone. **Figure 1** is a simplified diagram of all the players. Microbiota and Diet have a great influence on incretin action and glycemic control but SCFA, incretins, and insulin all have direct effects on the deposition of fat in adipocytes. Not listed in **Figure 1** is that glucose itself can be synthesized into fats. Incretins can affect glucsose metabolism by turning glucose into fats especially when the insulin levels are high.

Grant support

United States Department of Agriculture (USDA) Award #2021-38424-34955

Author details

Steven Coon
Department of Health and Environmental Sciences, Fort Peck Community College, Poplar, MT, USA

*Address all correspondence to: scoon@fpcc.edu

References

[1] Robertson MD, Jackson KG, Williams CM, Fielding BA, Frayn KN. Prolonged effects of modified sham feeding on energy substrate mobilization. The American Journal of Clinical Nutrition. 2001;**73**(1):111-117

[2] Servan PR. Obesity and diabetes. Nutrition in Hospital. 2013;**28**:138-143

[3] Piche ME, Tchernof A, Despres JP. Obesity phenotypes, diabetes, and cardiovascular diseases. Circulation Research. 2020;**126**(11):1477-1500

[4] Lim JZM, Ng NSL, Thomas C. Prevention and treatment of diabetic foot ulcers. Journal of the Royal Society of Medicine. 2017;**110**(3):104-109

[5] Beckman JA, Creager MA, Libby P. Diabetes and athersclerosis. Journal of the American Medical Association. 2002;**287**:2570-2581

[6] Shah MS, Brownlee M. Molecular and cellular mechanisms of cardiovascular disorders in diabetes. Circulation Research. 2016;**118**(11):1808-1829

[7] Perez-Panero AJ, Ruiz-Munoz M, Cuesta-Vargas AI, Gonzalez-Sanchez M. Prevention, assessment, diagnosis and management of diabetic foot based on clinical practice guidelines: A systematic review. Medicine (Baltimore). 2019;**98**(35):e16877

[8] Grennan D. Diabetic foot ulcers. Journal of the American Medical Association. 2019;**321**(1):114

[9] van Battum P, Schaper N, Prompers L, Apelqvist J, Jude E, Piaggesi A, et al. Differences in minor amputation rate in diabetic foot disease throughout Europe are in part explained by differences in disease severity at presentation. Diabetic Medicine. 2011;**28**(2):199-205

[10] Volmer-Thole M, Lobmann R. Neuropathy and diabetic foot syndrome. International Journal of Molecular Science. 2016;**17**(6):917

[11] Lim JZ, Ng NS, Thomas C. Prevention and treatment of diabetic foot ulcers. Journal of the Royal Society of Medicine. 2017;**110**(3):104-109

[12] Elliott TL, Pfotenhauer KM. Classification and diagnosis of diabetes. Primary Care. 2022;**49**(2):191-200

[13] Gurgel Penaforte-Saboia J, Couri CEB, Vasconcelos Albuquerque N, et al. Emerging roles of dipeptidyl peptidase-4 inhibitors in delaying the progression of Type 1 Diabetes Mellitus. Diabetes Metabolism Syndrome Obesity. 2021;**14**:565-573

[14] Wen L, Duffy A. Factors influencing the gut microbiota, inflammation, and Type 2 diabetes. The Journal of Nutrition. 2017;**147**(7):1468S-1475S

[15] Ma J, Li Z, Zhang W, Zhang C, Zhang Y, Mei H, et al. Comparison of the gut microbiota in healthy infants with different delivery modes and feeding types: A Cohort Study. Frontiers in Microbiology. 2022;**13**:868227

[16] Maselli DB, Camilleri M. Effects of GLP-1 and its analogs on gastric physiology in diabetes mellitus and obesity. Advances in Experimental Medicine and Biology. 2021;**1307**:171-192

[17] Holst JJ, Rosenkilde MM. GIP as a Therapeutic Target in Diabetes and Obesity: Insight From Incretin

Co-agonists. Journal of Clinical Endocrinology Metabolism. 2020;**105**:2710-2716

[18] Killion EA, Wang J, Yie J, Shi SD, Bates D, Min X, et al. Anti-obesity effects of GIPR antagonists alone and in combination with GLP-1R agonists in preclinical models. Science Translational Medicine. 2018;**10**:3392

[19] Norregaard PK, Deryabina MA, Tofteng Shelton P, Fog JU, Daugaard JR, Eriksson PO, et al. A novel GIP analogue, ZP4165, enhances glucagon-like peptide-1-induced body weight loss and improves glycaemic control in rodents. Diabetes, Obesity & Metabolism. 2018;**20**(1):60-68

[20] Killion EA, Lu SC, Fort M, Yamada Y, Veniant MM, Lloyd DJ. Glucose-dependent insulinotropic polypeptide receptor therapies for the treatment of obesity, Do Agonists = Antagonists? Endocrinology Review. 2020;**41**(1):1-21

[21] Miyawaki K, Yamada Y, Ban N, Ihara Y, Tsukiyama K, Zhou H, et al. Inhibition of gastric inhibitory polypeptide signaling prevents obesity. Nature Medicine. 2002;**8**(7):738-742

[22] Coon SD, Rajendran VM, Schwartz JH, Singh SK. Glucose-dependent insulinotropic polypeptide-mediated signaling pathways enhance apical PepT1 expression in intestinal epithelial cells. American Journal of Physiology. Gastrointestinal and Liver Physiology. 2015;**308**(1):G56-G62

[23] Coon SD, Schwartz JH, Rajendran VM, Jepeal L, Singh SK. Glucose-dependent insulinotropic polypeptide regulates dipeptide absorption in mouse jejunum. American Journal of Physiology. Gastrointestinal and Liver Physiology. 2013;**305**(10):G678-G684

[24] Veedfald S, Plamboeck A, Deacon CF, Hartmann B, Knop FK, Vilsboll T, et al. Cephalic phase secretion of insulin and other enteropancreatic hormones in humans. American Journal of Physiology. Gastrointestinal and Liver Physiology. 2016;**310**(1):G43-G51

[25] Lorentzen M, Madsbad S, Kehlet H, Tronier B. Effect of sham-feeding on glucose tolerance and insulin secretion. Acta Endocrinologica. 1987;**115**(1):84-86

[26] Teff KL. Cephalic phase pancreatic polypeptide responses to liquid and solid stimuli in humans. Physiology & Behavior. 2010;**99**(3):317-323

[27] Teff KL, Mattes RD, Engelman K. Cephalic phase insulin release in normal weight males: Verification and reliability. The American Journal of Physiology. 1991;**261**(4 Pt 1):E430-E436

[28] Hall KD, Farooqi IS, Friedman JM, Klein S, Loos RJF, Mangelsdorf DJ, et al. The energy balance model of obesity: Beyond calories in, calories out. The American Journal of Clinical Nutrition. 2022;**115**(5):1243-1254

[29] Ludwig DS, Aronne LJ, Astrup A, de Cabo R, Cantley LC, Friedman MI, et al. The carbohydrate-insulin model: A physiological perspective on the obesity pandemic. The American Journal of Clinical Nutrition. 2021:1873-1885

[30] Wallace AS, Chang AR, Shin JI, Reider J, Echouffo-Tcheugui JB, Grams ME, et al. Obesity and chronic kidney disease in US adults with Type 1 and Type 2 diabetes mellitus. The Journal of Clinical Endocrinology and Metabolism. 2022;**107**(5):1247-1256

[31] Rivas R, Dratz E, Wagner T, Secor G, Leckband A, Sands DC. Rapid Screening Methods of Potato Cultivars

for Low Glycemic Traits. BioRxiv. 2021. Submitted:1-27

[32] Gebeyew K, Chen K, Wassie T, Azad MAK, He J, Jiang W, et al. Dietary amylose/amylopectin ratio modulates cecal microbiota and metabolites in weaned goats. Frontiers in Nutrition. 2021;**8**:774766

[33] Xiao JB, Hogger P. Dietary polyphenols and type 2 diabetes: Current insights and future perspectives. Current Medicinal Chemistry. 2015;**22**(1):23-38

[34] Aryaeian N, Sedehi SK, Arablou T. Polyphenols and their effects on diabetes management: A review. Medical Journal of the Islamic Republic of Iran. 2017;**31**:134

[35] Vilarrasa N, San Jose P, Rubio MA, Lecube A. Obesity in patients with Type 1 diabetes: Links, risks and management challenges. Diabetes Metabolic Syndrome Obesity. 2021;**14**:2807-2827

[36] Thompson DR, Obarzanek E, Franko DL, Barton BA, Morrison J, Biro FM, et al. Childhood overweight and cardiovascular disease risk factors: The National Heart, Lung, and Blood Institute Growth and Health Study. The Journal of Pediatrics. 2007;**150**(1):18-25

[37] Bolla AM, Caretto A, Laurenzi A, Scavini M, Piemonti L. Low-carb and ketogenic diets in Type 1 and Type 2 diabetes. Nutrients. 2019;**11**(5):962

[38] Dabek A, Wojtala M, Pirola L, Balcerczyk A. Modulation of cellular biochemistry, epigenetics and metabolomics by ketone bodies. Implications of the ketogenic diet in the physiology of the organism and pathological states. Nutrients. 2020;**12**(3):788-802

[39] Bueno NB, de Melo IS, de Oliveira SL, da Rocha Ataide T. Very-low-carbohydrate ketogenic diet v. low-fat diet for long-term weight loss: A meta-analysis of randomised controlled trials. The British Journal of Nutrition. 2013;**110**(7):1178-1187

[40] de Cabo R, Mattson MP. Effects of intermittent fasting on health, aging, and disease. The New England Journal of Medicine. 2019;**381**(26):2541-2551

[41] Al Aamri KS, Alrawahi AH, Al Busaidi N, Al Githi MS, Al Jabri K, Al Balushi F, et al. The effect of low-carbohydrate ketogenic diet in the management of obesity compared with low caloric, low-fat diet. Clinical Nutrition ESPEN. 2022;**49**:522-528

[42] Leone A, De Amicis R, Battezzati A, Bertoli S. Adherence to the mediterranean diet and risk of metabolically unhealthy obesity in women: A Cross-Sectional Study. Frontiers in Nutrition. 2022;**9**:858206

[43] Ishikawa Y, Laing EM, Anderson AK, Zhang D, Kindler JM, Trivedi-Kapoor R, et al. Adherence to the dietary approaches to stop hypertension (DASH) diet is associated with low levels of insulin resistance among heart failure patients. Nutrition, Metabolism, and Cardiovascular Diseases. 2022:1841-1850

[44] Hirahatake KM, Jiang L, Wong ND, Shikany JM, Eaton CB, Allison MA, et al. Diet quality and cardiovascular disease risk in postmenopausal women with type 2 diabetes mellitus: The Women's Health Initiative. Journal of the American Heart Association. 2019;**8**(19):e013249

[45] Bach Knudsen KE. Microbial degradation of whole-grain complex carbohydrates and impact on short-chain fatty acids and health. Advances in Nutrition. 2015;**6**(2):206-213

[46] Verbeke KA, Boobis AR, Chiodini A, Edwards CA, Franck A, Kleerebezem M, et al. Towards microbial fermentation metabolites as markers for health benefits of prebiotics. Nutrition Research Reviews. 2015;**28**(1):42-66

[47] Morais CA, de Rosso VV, Estadella D, Pisani LP. Anthocyanins as inflammatory modulators and the role of the gut microbiota. The Journal of Nutritional Biochemistry. 2016;**33**:1-7

[48] Molinaro A, Bel Lassen P, Henricsson M, Wu H, Adriouch S, Belda E, et al. Imidazole propionate is increased in diabetes and associated with dietary patterns and altered microbial ecology. Nature Communications. 2020;**11**(1):5881

[49] Baothman OA, Zamzami MA, Taher I, Abubaker J, Abu-Farha M. The role of Gut Microbiota in the development of obesity and Diabetes. Lipids in Health and Disease. 2016;**15**:108

[50] Albenberg LG, Wu GD. Diet and the intestinal microbiome: Associations, functions, and implications for health and disease. Gastroenterology. 2014;**146**(6):1564-1572

[51] Galipeau HJ, Verdu EF. Gut microbes and adverse food reactions: Focus on gluten related disorders. Gut Microbes. 2014;**5**(5):594-605

[52] Macfarlane S, Macfarlane GT, Cummings JH. Review article: Prebiotics in the gastrointestinal tract. Alimentary Pharmacology & Therapeutics. 2006;**24**(5):701-714

[53] Zaman M, Chin K, Rai V, Majid H. Fiber and prebiotic supplementation in enteral nutrition: A systematic review and meta-analysis. World Journal of Gastroenterology. 2015;**17**:5372-5381

[54] Rajendran VM, Binder HJ. Apical membrane Cl-butyrate exchange: Mechanism of short chain fatty acid stimulation of active chloride absorption in rat distal colon. The Journal of Membrane Biology. 1994;**141**(1):51-58

[55] Morrison DJ, Preston T. Formation of short chain fatty acids by the gut microbiota and their impact on human metabolism. Gut Microbes. 2016;**7**(3):189-200

[56] Manokas T, Fromkes JJ, Sundaram U. Effect of chronic inflammation on ileal short-chain fatty acid/bicarbonate exchange. American Journal of Physiology. Gastrointestinal and Liver Physiology. 2000;**278**(4):G585-G590

[57] Wong C, Harris PJ, Ferguson LR. Potential benefits of dietary fibre intervention in inflammatory bowel disease. International Journal of Molecular Sciences. 2016;**17**(6):919

[58] Frank DN, St Amand AL, Feldman RA, Boedeker EC, Harpaz N, Pace NR. Molecular-phylogenetic characterization of microbial community imbalances in human inflammatory bowel diseases. Proceedings of the National Academy of Sciences of the United States of America. 2007;**104**(34):13780-13785

[59] Selkrig J, Wong P, Zhang X, Pettersson S. Metabolic tinkering by the gut microbiome: Implications for brain development and function. Gut Microbes. 2014;**5**(3):369-380

[60] Blaut M. Gut microbiota and energy balance: Role in obesity. The Proceedings of the Nutrition Society. 2015;**74**(3):227-234

[61] Macia L, Tan J, Vieira AT, Leach K, Stanley D, Luong S, et al. Metabolite-sensing receptors GPR43 and GPR109A facilitate dietary fibre-induced gut

homeostasis through regulation of the inflammasome. Nature Communications. 2015;**6**:6734

[62] Daly K, Cuff MA, Fung F, Shirazi-Beechey SP. The importance of colonic butyrate transport to the regulation of genes associated with colonic tissue homoeostasis. Biochemical Society Transactions. 2005;**33**(Pt 4): 733-735

[63] Daly K, Shirazi-Beechey SP. Microarray analysis of butyrate regulated genes in colonic epithelial cells. DNA and Cell Biology. 2006;**25**(1):49-62

[64] Bultman SJ. Interplay between diet, gut microbiota, epigenetic events, and colorectal cancer. Molecular Nutrition & Food Research. 2016:1-12

[65] Toden S, Lockett TJ, Topping DL, Scherer BL, Watson EJ, Southwood JG, et al. Butyrylated starch affects colorectal cancer markers beneficially and dose-dependently in genotoxin-treated rats. Cancer Biology & Therapy. 2014;**15**(11):1515-1523

[66] Rios-Covian D, Ruas-Madiedo P, Margolles A, Gueimonde M, de Los Reyes-Gavilan CG, Salazar N. Intestinal short chain fatty acids and their link with diet and human health. Frontiers in Microbiology. 2016;**7**:185

[67] Donohoe DR, Garge N, Zhang X, Sun W, O'Connell TM, Bunger MK, et al. The microbiome and butyrate regulate energy metabolism and autophagy in the mammalian colon. Cell Metabolism. 2011;**13**(5):517-526

[68] Sawzdargo M, George SR, Nguyen T, Xu S, Kolakowski LF, O'Dowd BF. A cluster of four novel human G protein-coupled receptor genes occurring in close proximity to CD22 gene on chromosome 19q13.1. Biochemical and Biophysical Research Communications. 1997;**239**(2):543-547

[69] Brown AJ, Goldsworthy SM, Barnes AA, Eilert MM, Tcheang L, Daniels D, et al. The Orphan G protein-coupled receptors GPR41 and GPR43 are activated by propionate and other short chain carboxylic acids. The Journal of biological chemistry. 2003;**278**(13):11312-11319

[70] Kuwahara A. Contributions of colonic short-chain Fatty Acid receptors in energy homeostasis. Frontier in Endocrinology (Lausanne). 2014;**5**:144

[71] Kaji I, Karaki S, Kuwahara A. Short-chain fatty acid receptor and its contribution to glucagon-like peptide-1 release. Digestion. 2014;**89**(1):31-36

[72] Kimura I, Inoue D, Hirano K, Tsujimoto G. The SCFA receptor GPR43 and energy metabolism. Frontiers in Endocrinology. 2014;**5**:85

[73] McNelis JC, Lee YS, Mayoral R, van der Kant R, Johnson AM, Wollam J, et al. GPR43 potentiates beta-cell function in obesity. Diabetes. 2015;**64**(9):3203-3217

[74] Sun M, Wu W, Liu Z, Cong Y. Microbiota metabolite short chain fatty acids, GPCR, and inflammatory bowel diseases. Journal of Gastroenterology. 2016:1-8

[75] Pereira MA, Pins JJ. Dietary fiber and cardiovascular disease: Experimental and epidemiologic advances. Current Atherosclerosis Reports. 2000;**2**(6):494-502

[76] Harris K, Kassis A, Major G, Chou CJ. Is the gut microbiota a new factor contributing to obesity and its metabolic disorders? Journal of Obesity. 2012;**2012**:879151

[77] Wu T, Tang Q, Yu Z, Gao Z, Hu H, Chen W, et al. Inhibitory effects of sweet cherry anthocyanins on the obesity development in C57BL/6 mice. International Journal of Food Sciences and Nutrition. 2014;**65**(3):351-359

[78] Trompette A, Gollwitzer ES, Yadava K, Sichelstiel AK, Sprenger N, Ngom-Bru C, et al. Gut microbiota metabolism of dietary fiber influences allergic airway disease and hematopoiesis. Nature Medicine. 2014;**20**(2):159-166

[79] Patterson E, Cryan JF, Fitzgerald GF, Ross RP, Dinan TG, Stanton C. Gut microbiota, the pharmabiotics they produce and host health. The Proceedings of the Nutrition Society. 2014;**73**(4):477-489

[80] Ojo O, Feng QQ, Ojo OO, Wang XH. The role of dietary fibre in modulating gut microbiota dysbiosis in patients with type 2 diabetes: A Systematic Review and Meta-Analysis of Randomised Controlled Trials. Nutrients. 2020;**12**(11)

[81] Duncan SH, Lobley GE, Holtrop G, Ince J, Johnstone AM, Louis P, et al. Human colonic microbiota associated with diet, obesity and weight loss. International Journal of Obesity. 2008;**32**(11):1720-1724

[82] Schwiertz A, Taras D, Schafer K, Beijer S, Bos NA, Donus C, et al. Microbiota and SCFA in lean and overweight healthy subjects. Obesity (Silver Spring). 2010;**18**(1):190-195

[83] Cheung SG, Goldenthal AR, Uhlemann AC, Mann JJ, Miller JM, Sublette ME. Systematic review of gut microbiota and major depression. Frontiers in Psychiatry. 2019;**10**:34

[84] Hu S, Wang Y, Lichtenstein L, Tao Y, Musch MW, Jabri B, et al. Regional differences in colonic mucosa-associated microbiota determine the physiological expression of host heat shock proteins. American Journal of Physiology. Gastrointestinal and Liver Physiology. 2010;**299**(6):G1266-G1275

[85] Liu T, Wang C, Wang YY, Wang LL, Ojo O, Feng QQ, et al. Effect of dietary fiber on gut barrier function, gut microbiota, short-chain fatty acids, inflammation, and clinical outcomes in critically ill patients: A systematic review and meta-analysis. JPEN Journal of Parenteral and Enteral Nutrition. 2021

[86] Fu X, Liu Z, Zhu C, Mou H, Kong Q. Nondigestible carbohydrates, butyrate, and butyrate-producing bacteria. Critical Review in Food Science and Nutrition. 2019;**59**(suppl. 1):S130-S152

[87] Hor PK, Pal S, Mondal J, Halder SK, Ghosh K, Santra S, et al. Antiobesity, antihyperglycemic, and antidepressive potentiality of rice fermented food through modulation of intestinal microbiota. Frontiers in Microbiology. 2022;**13**:794503

[88] Singh RK, Chang HW, Yan D, Lee KM, Ucmak D, Wong K, et al. Influence of diet on the gut microbiome and implications for human health. Journal of Translational Medicine. 2017;**15**(1):73

[89] Long J, Cai Q, Steinwandel M, Hargreaves MK, Bordenstein SR, Blot WJ, et al. Association of oral microbiome with type 2 diabetes risk. Journal of Periodontal Research. 2017;**52**(3):636-643

[90] Shin NR, Whon TW, Bae JW. Proteobacteria: Microbial signature of dysbiosis in gut microbiota. Trends in Biotechnology. 2015;**33**(9):496-503

[91] Fan Y, Han W. el al, Abnormal gut microbiota composition contributes

to the development of type 2 diabetes mellitus in db/db mice. Aging. 2019;**11**(22):10454-10467

[92] Stojanov S, Berlec A, Strukelj B. The influence of probiotics on the firmicutes/bacteroidetes ratio in the treatment of obesity and inflammatory bowel disease. Microorganisms. 2020;**8**(11)

[93] MacGregor G, Smith AJ, Thakker B, Kinsella J. Yoghurt biotherapy: Contraindicated in immunosuppressed patients? Postgraduate Medical Journal. 2002;**78**(920):366-367

[94] Moudgil V, Rana R, Tripathi PK, Farooq U, Sehgal R, Khan MA. Coprevalence of parasitic infections and diabetes in Sub-Himalayan region of Northern India. International Journal of Health Science (Qassim). 2019;**13**(1):19-24

[95] Yan LH, Mu B, Pan D, Shi YN, Yuan JH, Guan Y, et al. Association between small intestinal bacterial overgrowth and beta-cell function of type 2 diabetes. The Journal of International Medical Research. 2020;**48**(7):300060520937866

[96] Feng X, Li XQ. The prevalence of small intestinal bacterial overgrowth in diabetes mellitus: A systematic review and meta-analysis. Aging (Albany NY). 2022;**14**(2):975-988

[97] Hosseininasab Nodoushan SA, Nabavi A. The interaction of *Helicobacter pylori* Infection and Type 2 Diabetes Mellitus. Advanced Biomedical Research. 2019;**8**:15

[98] Chen B, Wang Z, Wang J, Su X, Yang J, Zhang Q, et al. The oral microbiome profile and biomarker in Chinese type 2 diabetes mellitus patients. Endocrine. 2020;**68**(3):564-572

[99] Matsha TE, Prince Y, Davids S, Chikte U, Erasmus RT, Kengne AP, et al. Oral microbiome signatures in diabetes mellitus and periodontal disease. Journal of Dental Research. 2020;**99**(6):658-665

[100] Pociot F, McDermott MF. Genetics of type 1 diabetes mellitus. Genes and Immunity. 2002;**3**(5):235-249

[101] Waters JL, Ley RE. The human gut bacteria Christensenellaceae are widespread, heritable, and associated with health. BMC Biology. 2019;**17**(1):83

[102] Goodrich JK, Waters JL, Poole AC, Sutter JL, Koren O, Blekhman R, et al. Human genetics shape the gut microbiome. Cell. 2014;**159**(4):789-799

Chapter 6

Targeting Matrix Metallopeptidase 9 (MMP-9) and Role of Quorum Sensing (QS) in Diabetic Foot Ulcers

Wakuma Wakene Jifar

Abstract

Diabetes-related foot ulcers (DFU) are a serious public health issue, and one of the main causes of death for diabetics is foot ulcers. Matrix metalloproteinase are crucial to both the pathophysiology of wounds and the healing process. MMPs have not previously been a focus for the treatment of DFUs due to the difficulty in differentiating between active MMPs and the two catalytically inactive forms of MMPs and the clinical failure of broad-spectrum MMP inhibitors in cancer. Managing bacterial infections by focusing on this quorum sensing (QS)-regulated process different from other management strategies. Despite the fact that the medical community has a thorough grasp of diabetic foot ulcers, research is continuously being done to find the most effective treatment for this crippling condition that is also safe to provide. Diabetic foot ulcers are brought on by a variety of factors, so a combination of therapies rather than a single medication will be the most effective course of treatment. This book chapter discusses the identification of active MMP-9 as the molecular cause of the diabetic wounds' resistance to healing as well as the unique therapeutic strategy of inhibiting this proteinase and about role of inhibiting the quorum sensing (QS) system in the treatment of diabetic foot ulcer.

Keywords: diabetic foot ulcer, quorum sensing (QS) system and targeting matrix metallopeptidase-9 (MMP-9), antimicrobial peptide

1. Introduction

A chronic metabolic condition called diabetes mellitus (DM) is characterized by hyperglycemia [1]. Defining diabetic foot (DF) as "the foot of a diabetic patient who has the potential risk of pathologic consequences including infection, ulceration, and/or destruction of deep tissues associated with neurologic abnormalities, various degrees of peripheral vascular disease, and/or metabolic complications of diabetes in the lower limb," according to the World Health Organization [2]. To prevent the onset of foot ulcers, early identification of the at-risk foot should be given top clinical attention [3]. Wound healing can be negatively impacted by stress and a steroid hormone called cortisol is high during times of stress and chronic inflammation and slows the healing of wounds. The inability of diabetic foot ulcers (DFU) to heal has been reported to be substantially correlated with CYP11B1, the enzyme that catalyzes cortisol production [4]. Cortisol levels have been linked to elevated MMP-9 levels in patients with coronary artery disease, and MMP-9 is reported to be induced and cortisol production stimulated by prostaglandin E2. The enhanced activity of matrix metalloproteinase (MMPs) is one of the causes of the resistance [5]. In 1960, the family of zinc-dependent endopeptidases known as MMPs was initially identified in tadpoles. Humans have 24 distinct MMPs that have a variety of substrates and roles [6]. MMPs are categorized in part according to the substrates they prefer to break down, including the gelatinases (MMP-2 and MMP-9), collagenases (MMP-1, MMP-8, and MMP-13), and stromelysins (MMP-3 and MMP-10) [7]. MMP expression and activity may be significantly impacted by DFU treatments that do not directly target MMPs. Most research has concentrated on the effects on MMP-9 in particular because it has long been thought that this proteinase has a role in wound healing. These investigations definitely showed that MMP-9 plays a negative effect in DFU healing, while MMP-8 plays a positive role. Approximately 15% of all diabetic patients get DFU, and of those, 84% have their lower limb amputated and 6% are hospitalized for gangrene and infections that are primarily caused by multidrug-resistant (MDR) microorganisms [8]. These pathogens include *Morganella morganii*, *Klebsiella pneumoniae*, *Proteus mirabilis*, *Streptococcus agalactiae*, *Streptococcus pyogenes*, *Streptococcus mitis*, *Staphylococcus aureus*, and *Enterococcus faecalis*, which dominate and populate the foot ulcer [9]. These pathogens exhibit virulence traits such biofilm formation and others, making antibiotic therapy ineffective against them. When bacterial colonies known as biofilms reach a certain size, they coordinate changes in gene expression *via* coordinated cell-to-cell communication (quorum sensing) and prepare to express additional virulent factors [10]. The development of biofilm on the skin surface of DFU is a further issue. And in DFU, biofilm is a crucial stage in the pathophysiology and it may delay recovery. Both MDR bacteria and microorganisms that produce biofilms create antibiotic-resistant conditions that cause the lesion to become chronic, infect, and, in the worst case, necessitate lower limb amputation. Managing bacterial infections by focusing on this quorum sensing (QS)-regulated process offers a novel strategy [11]. This book chapter discusses the identification of active MMP-9 as the molecular cause of the diabetic wounds' resistance to healing as well as the unique therapeutic strategy of inhibiting enzyme proteinase and about role of inhibiting the quorum sensing (QS) system in the treatment of diabetic foot ulcer.

2. Epidemiology

A diabetic person may have a 25% lifetime risk of developing a foot ulcer and diabetes, and patients experience lower limb amputations 15 times more frequently than non-diabetics. Diabetic foot ulcer had a 6.3% global prevalence, with type 2 diabetes having a higher prevalence than type 1 diabetes (6.4 and 5.5%), respectively. The country with the highest prevalence is Belgium (14.8%), followed by Canada and the US (13.0%). Of all the continents, North America has the highest frequency (13%) by far. Asia accounted for 5.5%, Europe for 5.1%, and Africa for 7.2% [12].

From different parts of Ethiopia, Addis Abeba, Jimma, Gondar, Bahir Dar, Mekele, Arbeminch, and Dessie have higher rates of diabetic foot ulcers than other major cities (1.36%, 25.76%, 13.62%, 21.22%, 12.28%, 14.87%, and 1.85%, respectively), according to a study by Tolossa et al. [13] and Degu et al [6].

3. Etiology and risk factors

Peripheral neuropathy and peripheral arterial disease are the most frequent causes of diabetic foot ulcers out of a range of interrelated factors. Diabetic foot ulcer is hence frequently referred to as neuropathic, neuroischemic, or ischemic ulcers. Since the 1990s, ischemic and neuroischemic ulcers have become the most common cause of diabetic foot ulcer, accounting for more than one-third of all cases [14, 15]. This is most likely due to increased awareness of the importance of ischemia in diabetic foot ulcer and its detrimental effects, but it may also be related to improved diagnostic procedures, which could have an impact on recommendations for diagnostic criteria [15, 16]. Between 70 and 83% of diabetic patients with serious soft-tissue infections have polymicrobial at the time of diagnosis [17]. Additionally, chronic diabetic foot ulcer has abnormally high matrix metalloprotease (MMP) levels compared with acute wounds, which promotes tissue disintegration and eventually impedes normal healing processes [18]. Diabetes and long-term smoking both raise the risk of gangrene [19]. Gas gangrene, a rare consequence of diabetic foot ulcers, can occur in people with these persistent non-healing lesions [20]. Gangrene is induced by a decrease in blood flow to the affected tissues, which causes a hypoxic environment and cellular damage from Advanced Glycation End Products, which leads to cell death [21]. Diabetes mellitus (DM) affects wound closure processes, beginning with a reduction in fibrinolysis and an imbalance of cytokines, which produces a change in wound closure [22]. Inadequate re-epithelialization is caused by hyperglycemia, which also inhibits angiogenesis and cell migration. Similarly, inadequate extracellular matrix (ECM) formation by fibroblasts contributes to the issue of inadequate wound healing [23, 24].

4. Issues with the present diabetic foot ulcer treatment

The primary treatment problems associated with diabetic foot ulcer are believed to be diabetic foot infections and delayed wound healing [25]. The idea of probiotic consumption is intriguing and significant in light of the growing concerns about antimicrobial drug resistance around the world because probiotics have the ability to strengthen the immune system and have anti-inflammatory properties, which may speed up the healing process after a wound [26]. World Health Organization estimates that 60% of microorganisms are developing resistance to important antibiotics and that all diseases will eventually develop 100% treatment resistance. Self-medication as well as ongoing administration of antibiotics could be one explanation for bacteria's increasing tolerance to them. Thorough study is still being done to find new ways to cure disorders brought on by these bacteria [27]. Probiotics and phage therapy are innovative techniques that can eliminate unwanted germs and possibly speed up the healing process [28].

5. The current strategy for managing diabetic foot ulcers

5.1 Antimicrobial peptides

Antimicrobial peptides (AMPs), which are present in almost all animals, are host defense peptides because they possess traits of both innate and adaptive immune systems. Short-polypeptide antimicrobial peptides called have a cationic characteristic and an amphipathic structure (usually no more than 60 amino acids). The majority of antimicrobial peptides operate as the first line of defense against a variety of pathogens, including bacteria, fungi, viruses, and protozoan parasites [29]. A recent analysis of publicly available patent data on the therapeutic use of antimicrobial peptides from 2003 to 2015 revealed that the majority of the claimed antimicrobial peptides were also described as the effective modulators of inflammation or neutralizers of pathogenic toxins in addition to being potent antibiotics [3, 30].

5.2 Growth factors

Platelet-derived growth factor, a mitogenic bioactive molecule, encourages undifferentiated mesenchymal cells to develop into mature tissue, which increases the production of new cells and speeds up wound healing. Additionally, platelets have the ability to promote angiogenesis and tissue migration from a preformed vascular bed. They can also provide vascular endothelial synthesis a final boost by inducing vasodilation [31].

5.3 Antidiabetic drugs and diabetic foot ulcers

5.3.1 Insulin

One of the most efficient methods of preventing diabetes problems is to maintain normoglycemia with enough meals and/or antidiabetic drugs. A reported 30.3% improvement in diabetic foot ulcer healing was seen after receiving insulin intravenously. A physiological glucose-lowering agent is known as insulin. Recently, there has been concern over the use of cutaneous insulin administration as a healing agent in diabetic foot ulcer [32, 33].

5.3.2 Dipeptidyl peptidase-4 (DPP-4) inhibitors

Dipeptidyl peptidase-4 is a significant enzyme that deactivates the cretin hormones glucagon-like peptide-1 and glucagon-like peptide. FDA-approved oral drugs known as 43 DPP-4 inhibitors for type II diabetes mellitus block dipeptidyl peptidase, improve the flow of infused hormones, and provide glycemic control as well as increased islet cell function. By reducing blood glucose levels, DPP-4 inhibitors including sitagliptin, vildagliptin, and anagliptin are used to treat diabetes. Exendin-4, a glucagon-like peptide-1 (GLP-1) receptor agonist derived from the saliva of the Gila monster, a large poisonous lizard found in the South Western region of the United States, was applied topically on experimental animals to speed up the healing of diabetic foot ulcer wounds whether or not adipose-derived stem cells were also present [34, 35].

5.4 Use of stem cells in diabetic foot ulcer

Diabetic foot ulcer can produce blood vessel and extracellular matrix cell precursors when stem cells, such as adipose-derived stem cells and endothelian progenitor cells, are introduced from bone marrow or other sources [36, 37]. To encourage the growth of new cells in the wound area, these progenitor cells can be injected into the wound [38].

5.5 Natural products

Aloe Vera, *Salvia miltiorrhiza*, *Mimosa tenuiflora*, *Alchemilla vulgaris*, *Angelica sinensis*, and *Moringa oleifera* are just a few of the plants utilized in a variety of cosmetic goods such as ointments, lotions, and gels. *M. oleifera* has been proven to drastically lower the levels of numerous cytokines, including but not limited to TNF-6, IL-6, and VEGF, as well as promote tissue granulation and reduce the size of diabetic foot ulcer wounds [39, 40]. Honey has healing, non-harmful antibacterial, antioxidant, and anti-inflammatory qualities that aid in the healing of burns and wounds. As an alternative therapy for diabetic foot ulcer, honey therapy has attracted a lot of interest in recent years and several studies have evaluated the effectiveness of honey therapy for treating diabetic foot ulcer at different stages [41, 42]. A recent study compared traditional saline solution dressings to honey dressings and found that the latter were more effective in terms of healing time and the number of lesions that were healed after 120 days [12, 43].

5.6 Bacteriophages

Bacteriophages are viruses that identify and reproduce in bacterial cells. Bacteriophages contain capsid protein heads that transport and protect the virus's genetic material [44]. The genetic material's size, organization (circular, linear, or segmented), and structure might change depending on the virus (ssDNA, dsDNA, ssRNA, dsRNA). Based on the bacteriophage used and the target proteins that aid in bacterial host attachment, bacteriophages are very host specific and will only attack specific strains [45]. Phages have so far been found to be successful in treating bacterial illnesses including cystic fibrosis, eye infections, new-born sepsis, urinary tract illnesses, and malignancies, in addition to skin infections brought on by bacteria like *P. aeruginosa*, *S. aureus*, *K. pneumoniae*, and *E. coli* [46]. According to Khalifa et al. [47] Myoviridae bacteriophage EFLK1 was successfully identified against the phage-resistant strain of Vancomycin-resistant *E. faecalis* V583 and due to genetic superiority, even phage-resistant bacteria can be eliminated by other phages from the same host in this research. According to El-Shibiny and El-Sahhar [48], bacteriophage T4 and the antibiotic cefotaxime can be used in combination to treat *E. coli* biofilms, although phage therapy can also be used on its own to clear them [49].

5.7 Probiotics therapy

One of these novel substances that is both commonly used and thoroughly researched for its potential to promote health is probiotics [50]. Probiotics are either a single strain or a combination of several organisms, and they have the power to improve wound healing after an inflammatory cell build-up at the wound site, boost immune systems, and produce anti-inflammatory action [19–26, 42–46, 49–51].

Recent randomized controlled trial experiments have demonstrated that certain intestinal bacteria, such as Lactobacillus and Bifidobacteria, inhibit cariogenic streptococci and Candida spp., and have positive effects on their oral action [52].

5.8 Amputation

For patients with infected diabetic foot ulcer and peripheral artery disease, amputation above the ankle is commonly an issue or requirement. Up to 60% of diabetics die within 5 years of having an amputation, which is higher than the mortality rate for other malignancies [52]. A diabetic foot ulcer specialist team should assess patients one to three times each month, especially those who are at high risk for ulceration and those who have undergone an amputation for a diabetic foot ulcer. Every time a patient comes in, their feet should be checked to see whether a vascular examination is necessary [53].

6. Novel treatment options for diabetic foot ulcers

6.1 Role of quorum sensing (QS) mechanism in inhibiting wound healing

The quorum sensing system is a two-part system made up of an enzyme that catalyzes the synthesis of the signal molecule (auto inducer) and a receptor molecule that binds to the signal molecule (such as acyl-homoserine lactone and cyclic peptides) and controls the transcription of numerous genes in addition to the gene that encodes the signal molecule [54]. Because the bacterial quorum sensing system is required for biofilm development in chronic wounds, it is an important target for anti-biofilm treatment. Because the quorum sensing system is reliant on signaling by auto-inducer chemicals, blocking these would prevent coordinated virulence action. Gram-positive and Gram-negative bacteria have a wide range of quorum sensing systems [55]. The capacity of glyceryl trinitrate (GTN) to suppress quorum sensing-based biofilm development in *P. aeruginosa* burn infections was investigated [56]. The FDA has approved the antibacterial and wound-healing compound glyceryl trinitrate. When administered in ointments at a concentration of 0.15% to 0.3%, it is used to treat anal fissures and to suppress growth tonic *Candida albicans*. *P. aeruginosa* was observed to produce less biofilm when exposed to glyceryl trinitrate [5, 57].

6.2 Targeting matrix metallopeptidase 9 (MMP-9) in diabetic foot ulcers

Wound healing can be hampered by stress. Cortisol, a steroid hormone, is increased during stress and chronic inflammation, and it slows wound healing Elevated Matrix metallopeptidase-9 levels that have been linked to higher cortisol levels in individuals with coronary artery disease. Prostaglandin E2 has been shown to increase cortisol release and to activate matrix metallopeptidase-9 [58]. One of the causes of the recalcitrance is the increased activity of the enzyme matrix metalloproteinase (MMPs). The preferred substrates of MMPs, such as gelatinases (MMP-2 and MMP-9), collagenases (MMP-1, MMP-8, and MMP-13), and stromelysins, are characterized in a variety of ways (MMP-3 and MMP-10). A second generation of orally bioactive broad-spectrum inhibitors was created as a result of the first generation of MMPIs being broad-spectrum zinc chelators with low bioavailability [59]. The medication becaplermin Gelatinase activity was reduced, but collagenase activity was unaffected; active MMP-9 was reduced, while active MMP-8 was unaffected [60]. MMP expression and activity may be significantly impacted by diabetic foot ulcer treatments that do not directly target matrix metallopeptidase. Most researches have concentrated on the effects on this proteinase specifically since MMP-9 has long been of interest in wound healing [61].

7. Conclusion

Millions of people with diabetes struggle with diabetic foot ulcers, a serious consequence of diabetes. Despite the fact that the medical community has a thorough grasp of diabetic foot ulcers, research is continuously being done to find the most effective treatment for this crippling condition that is also safe to provide. Diabetic foot ulcers are brought on by a variety of factors, so a combination of therapies rather than a single medication will be the most effective course of treatment. The current challenges in treating diabetic foot ulcers are caused by bacterial resistance to the antibiotics now being used. Treatment options for diabetic foot ulcers include targeting matrix metallopeptidase-9 (MMP-9) and inhibiting the quorum sensing (QS) system has been emerged.

Acknowledgements

I am grateful to my beloved wife Lalise Tesfaye wakjira for strengthening me morally during writing this book.

Conflict of interest

The authors declare no conflict of interest.

Author details

Wakuma Wakene Jifar
Department of Pharmacy, College of Health Sciences, Mettu University, Mettu, Ethiopia

*Address all correspondence to: wakewakish05@gmail.com

References

[1] Ciemins EL, Coon PJ, Fowles JB, Min S-j. Beyond health information technology: Critical factors necessary for effective diabetes disease management. Journal of Diabetes Science and Technology. 2009;**3**(3):452-460

[2] Foot IWGotD. International Consensus on the Diabetic Foot and Practical Guidelines on the Management and Prevention of the Diabetic Foot. International Diabetes Federation: Amsterdam. Available from: www idf org/bookshop. 2007

[3] Revathi V. Risk factors associated with the development of diabetic foot ulcer among adult type 2 diabetes mellitus patients in a secondary care setting in Pathanamthitta district. SCTIMST. 2016;**9**:1-2

[4] Christian LM, Graham JE, Padgett DA, Glaser R, Kiecolt-Glaser JK. Stress and wound healing. Neuroimmunomodulation. 2006;**13**(5-6):337-346

[5] Lazaro J, Izzo V, Meaume S, Davies A, Lobmann R, Uccioli L. Elevated levels of matrix metalloproteinases and chronic wound healing: An updated review of clinical evidence. Journal of Wound Care. 2016;**25**(5):277-287

[6] Degu H, Wondimagegnehu A, Yifru YM, Belachew A. Is health related quality of life influenced by diabetic neuropathic pain among type II diabetes mellitus patients in Ethiopia? PLoS One. 2019;**14**(2):e0211449

[7] Gross J, Lapiere CM. Collagenolytic activity in amphibian tissues: A tissue culture assay. Proceedings of the National Academy of Sciences. 1962;**48**(6):1014-1022

[8] Beyaz S, Güler ÜÖ, Bağır GŞ. Factors affecting lifespan following below-knee amputation in diabetic patients. Acta Orthopaedica et Traumatologica Turcica. 2017;**51**(5):393-397

[9] Sadeghpour Heravi F, Zakrzewski M, Vickery K, Armstrong DG, Hu H. Bacterial diversity of diabetic foot ulcers: Current status and future prospectives. Journal of Clinical Medicine. 2019;**8**(11): 1935

[10] LaSarre B, Federle MJ. Exploiting quorum sensing to confuse bacterial pathogens. Microbiology and Molecular Biology Reviews. 2013;**77**(1):73-111

[11] Jiang Q, Chen J, Yang C, Yin Y, Yao K. Quorum sensing: A prospective therapeutic target for bacterial diseases. BioMed Research International. 2019; **2019**:2-3

[12] Ibrahim AM. Diabetic foot ulcer: Synopsis of the epidemiology and pathophysiology. International Journal of Diabetes and Endocrinology. 2018;**3**:23

[13] Tolossa T, Mengist B, Mulisa D, Fetensa G, Turi E, Abajobir A. Prevalence and associated factors of foot ulcer among diabetic patients in Ethiopia: A systematic review and meta-analysis. BMC Public Health. 2020;**20**(1):1-14

[14] Abbott CA, Vileikyte L, Williamson S, Carrington AL, Boulton AJ. Multicenter study of the incidence of and predictive risk factors for diabetic neuropathic foot ulceration. Diabetes Care. 1998;**21**(7):1071-1075

[15] Gershater M, Löndahl M, Nyberg P, Larsson J, Thörne J, Eneroth M, et al. Complexity of factors related to outcome of neuropathic and neuroischaemic/

ischaemic diabetic foot ulcers: A cohort study. Diabetologia. 2009;**52**(3):398-407

[16] Lipsky BA, Aragón-Sánchez J, Diggle M, Embil J, Kono S, Lavery L, et al. IWGDF guidance on the diagnosis and management of foot infections in persons with diabetes. Diabetes/Metabolism Research and Reviews. 2016;**32**:45-74

[17] Kalaivani C, Kuppusamy G, Karri VVSR. Simvastatin loaded polycaprolactone-collagen scaffolds for the treatment of diabetic foot ulcer. Research Journal of Pharmacy and Technology. 2019;**12**(6):2637-2644

[18] Baltzis D, Eleftheriadou I, Veves A. Pathogenesis and treatment of impaired wound healing in diabetes mellitus: New insights. Advances in Therapy. 2014;**31**(8):817-836

[19] Al Wahbi A. Autoamputation of diabetic toe with dry gangrene: A myth or a fact? Diabetes, Metabolic Syndrome and Obesity: Targets and Therapy. 2018;**11**:255

[20] Pichu S, Sathiyamoorthy J, Krishnamoorthy E, Umapathy D, Viswanathan V. Impact of the hypoxia inducible factor-1α (HIF-1α) pro582ser polymorphism and its gene expression on diabetic foot ulcers. Diabetes Research and Clinical Practice. 2015;**109**(3):533-540

[21] Gary Sibbald R, Woo KY. The biology of chronic foot ulcers in persons with diabetes. Diabetes/Metabolism Research and Reviews. 2008;**24**(S1):S25-S30

[22] Theoret C. Physiology of wound healing. Equine Wound Management. 2016;**1**:1-13

[23] Guo S, DiPietro LA. Factors affecting wound healing. Journal of Dental Research. 2010;**89**(3):219-229

[24] Gallagher KA, Liu Z-J, Xiao M, Chen H, Goldstein LJ, Buerk DG, et al. Diabetic impairments in NO-mediated endothelial progenitor cell mobilization and homing are reversed by hyperoxia and SDF-1α. The Journal of Clinical Investigation. 2007;**117**(5):1249-1259

[25] Sekhar MS, Unnikrishnan M, Vijayanarayana K, Rodrigues GS, Mukhopadhyay C. Topical application/formulation of probiotics: Will it be a novel treatment approach for diabetic foot ulcer? Medical Hypotheses. 2014;**82**(1):86-88

[26] Oelschlaeger TA. Mechanisms of probiotic actions–A review. International Journal of Medical Microbiology. 2010;**300**(1):57-62

[27] World Bank. Pulling Together to Beat Superbugs: Knowledge and Implementation Gaps in Addressing Antimicrobial Resistance. Washington, DC: World Bank; 2019

[28] Brüssow H, Hendrix RW. Phage genomics: Small is beautiful. Cell. 2002;**108**(1):13-16

[29] Ginsburg I, van Heerden PV, Koren E. From amino acids polymers, antimicrobial peptides, and histones, to their possible role in the pathogenesis of septic shock: A historical perspective. Journal of Inflammation Research. 2017;**10**:7

[30] Jin G, Weinberg A, editors. Human antimicrobial peptides and cancer. In: Seminars in Cell & Developmental Biology. United Kingdom: Elsevier; 2019

[31] Ma C, Hernandez MA, Kirkpatrick VE, Liang L-J, Nouvong AL, Gordon II. Topical platelet-derived growth factor vs placebo therapy of diabetic foot ulcers offloaded with windowed casts: A randomized, controlled trial. Wounds: A

Compendium of Clinical Research and Practice. 2015;**27**(4):83-91

[32] Lima MH, Caricilli AM, de Abreu LL, Araújo EP, Pelegrinelli FF, Thirone AC, et al. Topical insulin accelerates wound healing in diabetes by enhancing the AKT and ERK pathways: A double-blind placebo-controlled clinical trial. PLoS One. 2012;**7**(5):e36974

[33] Öhnstedt E, Lofton Tomenius H, Vågesjö E, Phillipson M. The discovery and development of topical medicines for wound healing. Expert Opinion on Drug Discovery. 2019;**14**(5):485-497

[34] Seo E, Lim JS, Jun J-B, Choi W, Hong I-S, Jun H-S. Exendin-4 in combination with adipose-derived stem cells promotes angiogenesis and improves diabetic wound healing. Journal of Translational Medicine. 2017;**15**(1):1-9

[35] Clark GC, Casewell NR, Elliott CT, Harvey AL, Jamieson AG, Strong PN, et al. Friends or foes? Emerging impacts of biological toxins. Trends in Biochemical Sciences. 2019;**44**(4):365-379

[36] Blumberg SN, Berger A, Hwang L, Pastar I, Warren SM, Chen W. The role of stem cells in the treatment of diabetic foot ulcers. Diabetes Research and Clinical Practice. 2012;**96**(1):1-9

[37] Owczarczyk-Saczonek A, Wociór A, Placek W, Maksymowicz W, Wojtkiewicz J. The use of adipose-derived stem cells in selected skin diseases (vitiligo, alopecia, and nonhealing wounds). Stem Cells International. 2017;**2017**:1-2

[38] Qin H, Zhu X, Zhang B, Zhou L, Wang W. Clinical evaluation of human umbilical cord mesenchymal stem cell transplantation after angioplasty for diabetic foot. Experimental and Clinical Endocrinology & Diabetes. 2016;**124**(08):497-503

[39] Muhammad AA, Arulselvan P, Cheah PS, Abas F, Fakurazi S. Evaluation of wound healing properties of bioactive aqueous fraction from Moringa oleifera Lam on experimentally induced diabetic animal model. Drug Design, Development and Therapy. 2016;**10**:5-6

[40] Chin C-Y, Ng P-Y, Ng S-F. *Moringa oleifera* standardised aqueous leaf extract-loaded hydrocolloid film dressing: *In vivo* dermal safety and wound healing evaluation in STZ/HFD diabetic rat model. Drug Delivery and Translational Research. 2019;**9**(2):453-468

[41] Ramirez-Acuña JM, Cardenas-Cadena SA, Marquez-Salas PA, Garza-Veloz I, Perez-Favila A, Cid-Baez MA, et al. Diabetic foot ulcers: Current advances in antimicrobial therapies and emerging treatments. Antibiotics. 2019;**8**(4):193

[42] Azzini E, Giacometti J, Russo GL. Antioxidant Phytochemicals at the Pharma-Nutrition Interface. New York: Hindawi; 2017

[43] Jull AB, Cullum N, Dumville JC, Westby MJ, Deshpande S, Walker N. Honey as a topical treatment for wounds. Cochrane Database of Systematic Reviews. 2015;**3**:5-6

[44] Salmond GP, Fineran PC. A century of the phage: Past, present and future. Nature Reviews Microbiology. 2015;**13**(12):777-786

[45] Reindel R, Fiore CR. Phage therapy: Considerations and challenges for development. Clinical Infectious Diseases. 2017;**64**(11):1589-1590

[46] Oliveira A, Sousa JC, Silva AC, Melo LD, Sillankorva S. Chestnut honey and bacteriophage application to control *Pseudomonas aeruginosa* and *Escherichia coli* biofilms: Evaluation in an ex vivo wound model. Frontiers in Microbiology. 2018;**9**:1725

[47] Khalifa L, Gelman D, Shlezinger M, Dessal AL, Coppenhagen-Glazer S, Beyth N, et al. Defeating antibiotic-and phage-resistant Enterococcus faecalis using a phage cocktail in vitro and in a clot model. Frontiers in Microbiology. 2018;**9**:326

[48] El-Shibiny A, El-Sahhar S. Bacteriophages: The possible solution to treat infections caused by pathogenic bacteria. Canadian Journal of Microbiology. 2017;**63**(11):865-879

[49] Gelman D, Beyth S, Lerer V, Adler K, Poradosu-Cohen R, Coppenhagen-Glazer S, et al. Combined bacteriophages and antibiotics as an efficient therapy against VRE *Enterococcus faecalis* in a mouse model. Research in Microbiology. 2018;**169**(9):531-539

[50] Jifar WW, Atnafie SA, Angalaparameswari S. A review: Matrix Metallopeptidase-9 nanoparticles targeted for the treatment of diabetic Foot ulcers. Journal of Multidisciplinary Healthcare. 2021;**14**:3321

[51] Lew LC, Liong MT. Bioactives from probiotics for dermal health: Functions and benefits. Journal of Applied Microbiology. 2013;**114**(5):1241-1253

[52] Malyar NM, Freisinger E, Meyborg M, Lüders F, Gebauer K, Reinecke H, et al. Amputations and mortality in in-hospital treated patients with peripheral artery disease and diabetic foot syndrome. Journal of Diabetes and its Complications. 2016;**30**(6):1117-1122

[53] Mavrogenis AF, Megaloikonomos PD, Antoniadou T, Igoumenou VG, Panagopoulos GN, Dimopoulos L, et al. Current concepts for the evaluation and management of diabetic foot ulcers. EFORT Open Reviews. 2018;**3**(9):513-525

[54] Brackman G, Coenye T. Quorum sensing inhibitors as anti-biofilm agents. Current Pharmaceutical Design. 2015;**21**(1):5-11

[55] Abbas HA, Shaldam MA. Glyceryl trinitrate is a novel inhibitor of quorum sensing in *Pseudomonas aeruginosa*. African Health Sciences. 2016;**16**(4):1109-1117

[56] Das L, Singh Y. Quorum sensing inhibition: A target for treating chronic wounds. In: Biotechnological Applications of Quorum Sensing Inhibitors. Berlin/Heidelberg, Germany: Springer; 2018. pp. 111-126

[57] Yousif A, Jamal MA, Raad I. Biofilm-based central line-associated bloodstream infections. Biofilm-Based Healthcare-Associated Infections. 2015;**10**:157-179

[58] Stojadinovic O, Gordon KA, Lebrun E, Tomic-Canic M. Stress-induced hormones cortisol and epinephrine impair wound epithelization. Advances in Wound Care. 2012;**1**(1):29-35

[59] Jones JI, Nguyen TT, Peng Z, Chang M. Targeting MMP-9 in diabetic foot ulcers. Pharmaceuticals. 2019;**12**(2):79

[60] Hariono M, Yuliani SH, Istyastono EP, Riswanto FD, Adhipandito CF. Matrix metalloproteinase 9 (MMP9) in wound healing of diabetic foot ulcer: Molecular target and structure-based drug design. Wound Medicine. 2018;**22**:1-13

[61] Greene AK, Puder M, Roy R, Arsenault D, Kwei S, Moses MA, et al. Microdeformational wound therapy: Effects on angiogenesis and matrix metalloproteinases in chronic wounds of 3 debilitated patients. Annals of Plastic Surgery. 2006;**56**(4):418-422

Chapter 7

Current Perspective of Prevention and Management of Diabetic Foot

Deephikaa Ramakrishnan Ramesh, Faiz Ahmed Shaikh and Muhammad Ilyas Nadeem

Abstract

Diabetes-related foot infections and ulcers are frequent complications of the condition. These problems are also frequent, cause significant discomfort, frequently come back, and lead to morbidity and mortality, placing a huge financial burden on the patient and society. To start and direct treatment, it is crucial to comprehend the role of important contributing factors such as diabetic neuropathy, peripheral arterial disease, and immune system dysfunction. Beginning with a comprehensive physical examination and detailed history, diabetic foot disease is managed. A thorough medical examination should pay particular attention to any indication of diabetic foot ulcers or infection, as well as the symptoms of peripheral vascular disease and diabetic neuropathy. Analgesics and antibiotics should be used for pain management and infection control respectively. A multidisciplinary strategy focusing on patient education should be incorporated into prevention measures.

Keywords: diabetic foot ulcer, pain management, infection control, patient education

1. Introduction

According to the International Diabetes Federation, diabetes is one of the twenty-first century's biggest global health emergencies and one of the top 10 causes of death worldwide [1]. Over the past 30 years, global prevalence has increased tremendously [2], and the trend is expected to continue to rise from the current 5.1 percent to 7.7 percent in 2030 [3]. Diabetes mellitus is a group of autoimmune, metabolic, and genetic illnesses that all have one thing in common which is hyperglycemia [4]. It is now becoming a major public health problem worldwide, putting unsustainable demands on individuals, caregivers, health systems, and society.

According to the WHO, officials throughout the world are concentrating their efforts on four non-communicable diseases (NCDs) that are recognized as being important public health issues. One of these diseases is diabetes. The prevalence of diabetes has considerably increased during the past few decades, as well as the number of cases [5].

Diabetes is becoming more and more prevalent, increasing the risk of complications. One of the most frightening effects of diabetes is foot disease. The term "Diabetic Foot" encompasses a number of conditions related to diabetes, including diabetic neuropathy, peripheral vascular disease, Charcot's neuroarthropathy, foot ulceration, osteomyelitis, and the possibility of limb amputation as a preventive outcome [6]. Diabetic foot is a terrible disability, requiring extended periods of time and is insurmountable, growing expenses, with the ever-present possibility of amputation. Diabetic foot ulcers, which are injuries to all layers of skin, necrosis, or gangrene that typically develop on the bottoms of the feet as a result of peripheral neuropathy or peripheral arterial disease, can occur in diabetic patients [7, 8].

1.1 Epidemiology of diabetic foot

Males and people over the age of 60 are more likely to develop diabetic foot problems. There is a dearth of reliable data on the prevalence and frequency of diabetic foot problems. According to current studies, the yearly happenings of diabetic foot ulcers in the generalized population is 1–4 percent, with a prevalence of 4–10 percent [6]. According to one study, diabetic foot problems account for 12% of all diabetes hospital admissions. In 2013, 11 percent of all diabetic patients admitted to a tertiary facility in East Coast Malaysia had significant limb amputation. Diabetics have a 12.3 times higher risk of amputation due to foot problems than the general population [9].

1.2 Etiology of diabetic foot

There are a few causes of diabetic foot ulcers.

1.2.1 Diabetic neuropathy

Diabetes neuropathy expresses itself through the motor, autonomic, and sensory components of the nervous system [10]. Diabetic neuropathy affects more than half of patients over the age of 60 and raises the risk of foot ulcers by sevenfold. Damage to the innervations of the intrinsic foot muscles leads to an imbalance in the foot's flexion and extension of the directly impacted foot. Anatomic foot malformations lead to abnormal bone prominences and pressure points, which lead to skin breakdown and ulceration over time [11]. The patient may be unaware of the toxic nature of neuropathy, along with the significance of routine diabetic foot assessment. Motor neuropathy causes foot ulceration which is caused by muscle atrophy, foot deformity, altered foot biomechanics, and pressure redistribution [6].

1.2.2 Peripheral vascular disease

Peripheral vascular disease. Although the peripheral vascular disease can occur at any level of the arterial tree, atheroma appears to prefer specific locations, specifically bifurcations and bends in the artery where hemodynamic shear stress is low or flow separation occurs. In the lower limb, the aortoiliac segment and the superficial femoral artery (SFA) in the adductor canal are common sites. Diabetics often include more distal vessels underneath the trifurcation, for example, the peroneal, anterior, and posterior tibias. Unexpectedly, vessels in the feet, such as the dorsalis pedis, are frequently spared [11].

1.2.3 Infection or injury

Due to certain anatomical peculiarities, a profound infection inside a diabetic foot is indeed a limb-threatening condition. The foot has several compartments that communicate with one another, enabling the infection to spread from one area to another and the patient's ability to continue ambulation, allowing the infection to spread even further [11]. On the other hand, patients with peripheral vascular disease who present with a minor injury may develop an excruciating and entirely ischaemic foot ulcer [12].

1.2.4 Immunopathy

Patients with type 2 diabetes have a significantly compromised immune system compared to otherwise healthy people. Diabetic foot infection is therefore a limb-threatening and debilitating disease. Increased blood glucose increases polymorphonuclear cell functions and hampers pro-inflammatory cytokines such as chemotaxis, adherence, phagocytosis, and intracellular killing [13]. The immune system is jeopardized by decreased leukocyte activity, an inappropriate inflammatory response, and disruption of cellular immunity [14].

1.2.5 Osteomyelitis

Osteomyelitis is caused by a profound soft tissue infection spreading continuously from the cortex towards the bone marrow. Osteomyelitis is related to the majority of deep, long-term foot infections. It can be difficult to diagnose osteomyelitis in a diabetic patient. It is difficult to distinguish soft tissue infectious disease from bone infection, as well as infectious diseases from non-infectious diseases [11].

2. Prevention and management of diabetic foot

2.1 Principles of management

The foremost is treating infections; secondly, to determine if any related ischaemia is revascularisable; thirdly, is to limit exertion to the area of ulceration; The fourth focus is to enhance the wound or ulcer's situation through wound-bed preparation, topical treatments, and callus removal. The avoidance of ulcer recurrence can be the focus once the wound has healed.

2.1.1 Debridement

Diabetic feet develop calluses as a result of frequent sheer force [15]. Debridement is known as a wound treatment that removes slough or scar tissue. This necrotic tissue works as a barrier, preventing wound edges from coming together; eliminating it allows wound healing [16]. To accomplish this function, the base of abnormal injuries, wound edge tissue such as epidermal hyperkeratosis (callus) and necrotic dermal tissue, debris, and bacterial elements which can hinder wound healing are removed. According to multiple clinical trial studies, debridement promotes the growth of granulation tissue, which aids in the healing of wounds [17, 18].

According to Frank et al. theory, because there is fresh wound bleeding at the time of debridement in diabetic foot ulcers, debridement can raise VEGF levels [19]. Debridement of diabetic foot ulcers on a regular basis may speed up wound healing, however, there is little evidence to back up this claim [20].

Clinical trials have shown that only surgical debridement is effective out of the 5 methods of debridement: enzymatic, autolytic, mechanical, and biologic.

Sharp debridement is used during surgery to remove all bone and dead tissue. Debridement's goal is to change the environment for chronic wound healing to one that is more conducive to acute wound healing. Enzymatic debridement uses enzymes that have been carefully formulated to break down proteins, including collagenase, trypsin, papain/urea from papaya, streptokinase as well as fibrinolysis/DNAse, and streptodornase combinations. Natural autolytic debridement occurs in ulcers that are healthy, moist, and perfused. Lavage, pressure irrigation, dry-wet dressing, and hydrotherapy are used for mechanical debridement. Utilizing the sterile Lucilia sericata fly larvae as the debridement method, in which the necrotic tissue is found to be able to be thinned out due to the proteolytic enzyme emitted by the larvae [21].

2.1.2 Offloading

'Offloading' solutions reduce pressure even more and redistribute weight-bearing load over a bigger region of the foot [15]. The most straightforward method is mandatory bed rest; however, this is ineffective due to poor compliance and the risk of consequences such as osteoporosis as well as deep vein thrombosis. Total contact casting (TCC) is evidence-based offloading as well as the best time-tested approach since it ensures compliance and reduces the bulk and weight of the cast. This relieves ulcer pressure and spreads throughout the foot, which causes wound healing to be faster [6]. This procedure enables the patient to move around while receiving therapy and is effective in reducing edema, which can impede wound healing. Even though difficult and time-consuming, TCC can alleviate the pressure upon that incision, as evidenced by 73–100% healing. The drawbacks of TCC include the need for time as well as skill, the potential for new injuries caused by plaster irritation, the difficulty of daily injury assessment, the increased usage of removable cast walkers, and the lack of daily wound examination, dressing changes, and infection detection. Additional techniques include bed rest, using wheelchairs, walkers, and shoes that are carefully made [22, 23].

2.1.3 Infection management

Patients' self-education, improved diabetes knowledge and understanding, and self-management activities improved prescription adherence to oral diabetic drugs in a case-controlled trial. Duloxetine and pregabalin are recommended as first-line pain relievers by the National Institute of Clinical Excellence [15].

The three components of ulcer management are callus removal, infection destruction, as well as decrease of forces of weight bearing, which frequently necessitates foot elevated bed rest. To reveal the ulcer's floor and enable effective drainage of the lesion, extra keratin should be removed using a scalpel blade. When there are lesions or an ulcer that is deep penetrating that does not heal or keeps coming back, a radiograph should be conducted to check for osteomyelitis [24].

After the callus has been removed, the bacterial swab has to be collected from the ulcer's floor; the excised tissue may produce even more trustworthy results. Patients with superficial ulcers can receive suitable oral antibiotics until the ulcer heals and be treated as outpatients. Staphylococci, streptococci, and occasionally anaerobes are the most common pathogens that can infect a superficial ulcer. Amoxicillin, flucloxacillin, and metronidazole are therefore used to begin treatment and are changed once bacteriological culture findings are obtained. Considerable knowledge and laboratory assistance are required for the selection and duration of antibiotic treatment [24]. A wound culture-based antibiotic regimen has also been shown to benefit diabetic foot ulcers with superadded infection [15]. Microorganism resistance should be considered while choosing a treatment. Microorganism resistance should be considered while choosing a treatment. Oral antibiotics with Gram-positive germ activity for minor infections [25] as well as antibiotics active on Gram-positive as well as Gram-negative bacteria, which includes anaerobic bacteria, for moderate to terribly severe infections [16].

Patients who exhibit any of the risk factors stated on and in the box should be sent to the hospital right away for prompt care and assessment. They need to stay in bed and immediately begin receiving intravenous antibiotics. It could be necessary to use an intravenous insulin pump to regulate blood glucose levels.

Antibiotics: Bacteriological cultures require a broad spectrum of antibiotic coverage within the first 24 hours. Quadruple therapy may include amoxicillin, flucloxacillin, metronidazole (for anaerobes), and either ceftazidime 1 g three times daily or gentamicin (for Gram-negative organisms). When the outcomes of the bacteriological culture are available, this treatment can be modified. Multiple resistant *Staphylococcus aureus* (MRSA) is a severe issue because, first, it can cause sepsis' devastating effects and, second, these individuals need isolation while in the hospital. Both intramuscular teicoplanin and intravenous vancomycin are available as therapies (**Figure 1**) [24].

Analgesics: Peripheral neuropathy, ischemia, and infection are the three main causes of pain in diabetic feet. With other painful conditions, the treatment is comparable. The WHO analgesic ladder suggests using straightforward analgesics for mild to moderate pain, for example, paracetamol or a non-steroidal anti-inflammatory drug.

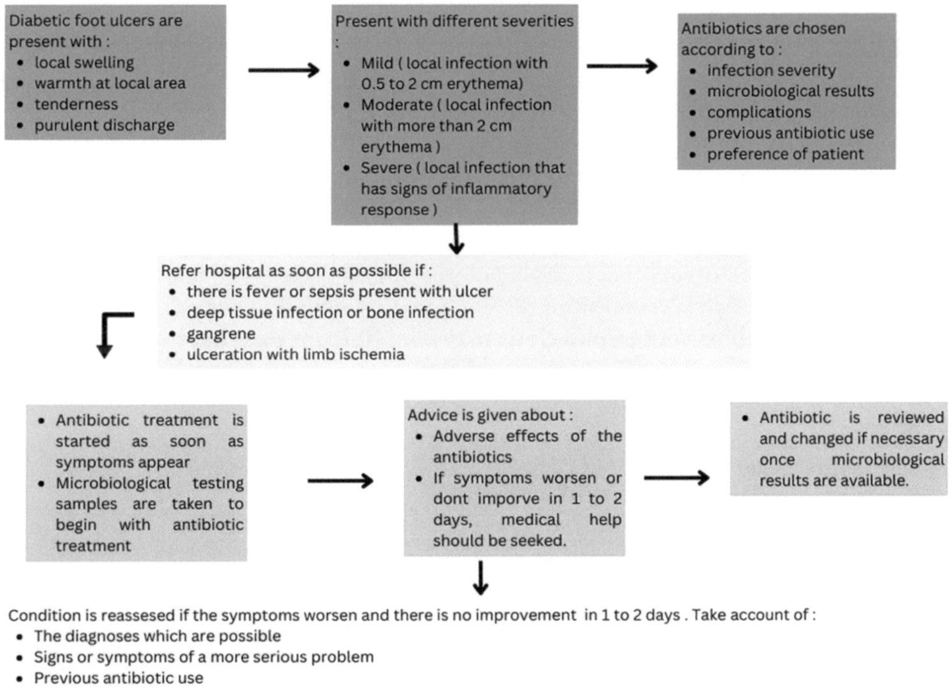

Figure 1.
Treatment algorithm for the diabetic foot. Note: From Ref. [26].

In moderate pain, additional mild opioids such as dihydrocodeine or tramadol should be taken into consideration. Patients experiencing moderate to severe pain should be given potent opioids, such as morphine. In neuropathic pain, adjuvants are used at all levels of the analgesic ladder. Adjuvants include, for instance, antidepressants like amitriptyline and anticonvulsants like duloxetine (e.g. gabapentin or pregabalin) (**Tables 1** and **2**).

Surgical debridement is required to flush pus and abscess cavities as well as remove all gangrenous and contaminated tissue, such as osteomyelitis-related devitalized and infected bone. It is advised to send deep tissue swabs to the lab. If necrosis has occurred in the digit, a ray amputation to remove the toe and a portion of its accompanying metatarsal is required in the neuropathic foot with intact circulation. In some cases, skin grafting is required to hasten wound healing [24].

2.1.4 Negative therapy wound pressure

Another increasingly popular technique for treating diabetic foot ulcers involves targeted negative pressure wound therapy, which basically involves draining wound fluid through a vacuum seal. In comparison to treating ulcers with a typical gauze dressing, this often involves a shorter treatment period and is intended to improve the perfusion of tissues and encourage the creation of granulation tissue. However, there is no found statistically significant difference (p 1/4 0.15) in the amount of time needed for wound closure between negative pressure wound therapy and the usual wound care from a Canadian evidence-based study [28].

2.1.5 Growth factors and skin substitutes

In a meta-analysis of the research supporting the use of active skin replacements as well as the growth factors in the treatment of diabetic foot ulcers, Buchberger et al. found that the combination of these treatments did lead to a greater incidence and quicker time to complete wound healing [29].

Recent research has also indicated that the administration of granulocyte colony-stimulating factor can reduce the need for surgical procedures, as seen by a general decline in the risk of amputation for diabetic foot ulcers. Granulocyte colony-stimulating factor boosts neutrophil activity by increasing the release of neutrophil progenitors from the bone marrow. More research is still needed to support these findings and determine which patient populations may benefit from this therapy the most.

Analgesics
Mild to moderate pain: • Paracetamol or non-steroidal anti-inflammatory drugs, Ibuprofen
Moderate pain: • Mild opioids such as dihydrocodeine or tramadol
Moderate to severe pain: • Morphine
Note: From Ref. [27].

Table 1.
Pain management in diabetic foot.

Mild infection	Moderate or Severe infection
First choice antibiotics: • Quadruple therapy • (Amoxicillin, Flucloxacillin, Metronidazole, and Ceftazidime 500 mg 1 g three times daily or gentamicin)	First choice antibiotics: Flucloxacillin with: • Oral: Flucloxacillin (1 g four times daily) with or without Gentamicin (5 to 7 mg/kg once daily IV) and/or Metronidazole (400 mg three times daily) • IV: Flucloxacillin (1 to 2 g four times daily) with or without Gentamicin (5 to 7 mg/kg once daily IV) and/or Metronidazole (500 mg three times daily) Co-trimoxazole with: • Oral: Co-trimoxazole (960 mg twice daily) with or without Gentamicin (5 to 7 mg/kg once daily) Metronidazole (400 mg three times daily) • IV: Co-trimoxazole (960 mg twice daily) with or without Gentamicin (5 to 7 mg/kg once daily) Metronidazole (500 mg three times daily) Ceftriaxone with: • Oral: Ceftriaxone (2 g once a day IV) with Metronidazole (400 mg three times daily) • IV: Ceftriaxone (2 g once a day IV) with Metronidazole (500 mg three times daily
Alternative oral antibiotic for patients with Penicillin allergy: • Clarithromycin (500 mg twice daily for 7 days) • Doxycycline (200 mg on the first day then continued to 100 mg once daily for 7 days)	Additional antibiotics if Pseudomonas aeruginosa is detected or confirmed: • Piperacillin with tazobactam (4.5 g three times a day IV) Clindamycin with: • Oral: Clindamycin (150 to 300 mg four times daily) with Ciprofloxacin (500 mg twice daily) and/or Gentamicin 5 to 7 mg once daily IV • IV: Clindamycin (600 mg to 2.7 g daily IV in two to four divided doses) with Ciprofloxacin (400 mg twice or thrice daily) and/or Gentamicin 5 to 7 mg once daily IV
Alternative oral antibiotic for pregnant patients with Penicillin allergy • Erythromycin (500 mg four times daily for 7 days)	Additional antibiotics if MRSA is detected or confirmed: • Vancomycin (15 to 20 mg/kg twice or thrice daily IV) • Teicoplanin (6 mg/kg 12 hourly for three doses then 6 mg/kg once daily)

Table 2.
Infection control with antibiotics in diabetic foot.

2.1.6 Glycaemic control

In patients with insulin-dependent diabetes mellitus, increasing evidence shows that strict glycemic control prevents and slows the progression of diabetic retinopathy, nephropathy, and neuropathy. It is important for diabetic patients to maintain a proper glycemic index to avoid any further complications such as the diabetic foot.

2.1.7 Dressing

A dressing is a substance that is applied topically to the area to help the wound heal and protect it. Plaster serves as a barrier between the dressing and the wound, preventing direct dressing contact. Film, hydrogel, composite, alginate, hydrocolloid, foam, and other absorptive dressings including negative pressure wound therapy are some of the several types of dressings (NPWT) [18].

The primary function of a closed-clean wound or granulated wound is to create a moist healing environment that promotes cell migration and protects against dry sores. The type and quantity of exudate present in the wound determine the appropriate dressing. Cuts with a little amount of exudate are ideally suited for hydrogel dressing, film, and composite use. Hydrocolloids are utilized for wounds with exudate amounts, and alginate, foam, and NPWT are frequently used for wounds with exudate amounts. Before applying a dressing, injuries with significant necrotic tissue should be debrided [18].

A sponge which is put on the wound, covering it with a dressing which is airtight, and then installing a vacuum is known as negative pressure wound therapy or closure of wound with vacuum. Large lymphatic leaks and fistulas can be treated using negative pressure wound therapy. The primary goal of NPWT is to reduce edema; by removing lymphatic or interstitial fluid, it increases the passage of interstitial oxygen into cells. The MMP enzymes and collagenase, in which of levels rise in chronic wounds, are also eliminated by negative pressure wound therapy [18].

2.2 Prevention of diabetic foot

2.2.1 Primary prevention

Reduced cardiovascular risks make the foot less susceptible to ischemia caused by macrovascular disease, while improved blood-glucose control reduces microvascular consequences. Patients' feet that are at risk will be identified by routine surveillance, and they should undergo specialized care.

2.2.1.1 Metabolic control

Hyperglycemia enhances the macrovascular and microvascular problems in diabetes. Foot ulcerations that can result in limb amputations are linked to this higher risk.

A systematic review comparing intense control (HbA1c (HbA1c) 6–7.5%) with less intensive glycemic control found a lower risk of amputees (RR = 0.65, 95% CI 0.45 to 0.94) and a delayed decline in sensory vibration cutoff point (MD = -8.27, 95% CI -9.75 to −6.79). Other neuropathic shifts (RR = 0.89, 95% CI 0.75 to 1.05) and ischemic changes (RR = 0.92, 95% CI 0.67 to1.26), on the other hand, were unaffected [30].

In a Cochrane literature review on the prevention of diabetes-related neuropathy, focused blood glucose control (HbA1c 7.0%) significantly reduced the risk of continuing to develop neuropathy in T1DM however not in T2DM at 12 months follow-up. However, including both T1DM and T2DM, this was associated with a higher risk of severe hypoglycemia, excess weight, hospital admissions, and deaths [32] (**Figure 2**).

2.2.1.2 Preventive footcare

Walking or having to stand while structurally trying to load the feet exemplifies stress on the plantar surface, exacerbating compression and shear stress. Foot abnormalities, such as hammer and claw toes, which are frequent in diabetic individuals, add to the pressure and tension. A systematic review of apparel and off-loading techniques throughout diabetics of neuropathy found that bespoke insoles reduced recurring metatarsal head ulcers at 15 months (p = 0.007) [33].

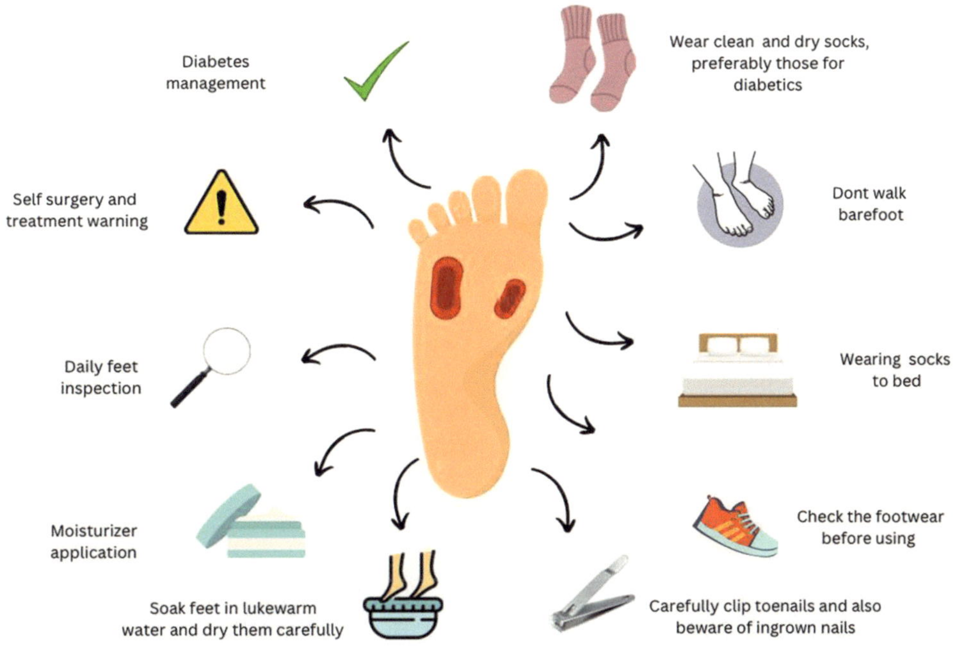

Figure 2.
Management of diabetic foot disease. Note: From Ref. [31].

- When worn more frequently than 80% of the time, made-to-order shoes with the plantar pressure drop reduced the prevalence of foot ulcers markedly (25.7% vs. 47.8%).
- When compared to ready-made footwear, intensive footwear therapy for diabetic patients with neuropathy, deformity, prior ulceration, and mild amputation dramatically reduced the first or recurrent ulcer.

2.2.2 Secondary prevention

A past lesion is a very good indicator of future ulceration. To prevent aberrant pressure loading, efforts should be made. These efforts may include cushioning for weak and immobile persons and specifically fitting footwear for mobile people, but such interventions must be correctly targeted. Foot care, individualized examination, routine podiatry, and the availability of emergency contact information should all be emphasized in education. Education reduced recurrent ulceration and amputation by three times in under 13 months for one trial, whilst McCabe and colleagues discovered a decrease in amputees but no change in fresh ulceration. Education also increases knowledge and behavior connected to sickness. These results need to be verified. If education efforts were primarily directed at professionals, they might be more successful [34].

2.2.2.1 Patient education

Because their bodies do not respond to pain normally, patients with neuropathy frequently overlook signals of harm. The patient's adherence to self-care will be impacted by this. In order to decrease diabetic foot issues, extensive education on adequate diabetic foot care is required. In preventing foot issues, knowledge of patients needs to be planned out and repeated at regular intervals. A doctor, podiatrist, or other trained healthcare professionals who dedicate time to explaining the fundamental care of the foot, callus, and nail can give patient education. Every year, this should be done [35].

The key to preventing ulcer formation is good foot care and management of minor foot injuries. The patient's overall foot inspection is the basis for good foot care. Gentle washing with detergent and water, accompanied by the usage of topical creams, aids in the preservation of healthy skin that is greater resistant to breakdown and injury. Minimal foot injuries and infections, such as cuts, scrapes, ulcers, and athlete's foot, can be unintentionally aggravated by home remedies that impede healing. Patients should be cautioned to avoid hot showers, heating pads, and harsh topical medications such as betadine, hydrogen peroxide, and iodine. Ulcers can be avoided by gently having to clean small cuts and applying a topical antibiotic to retain the site moist. In addition, any slight wound that does not heal quickly should be evaluated by a physician.

3. Conclusion

It takes careful coordination between numerous groups in primary care and hospital services to successfully manage diabetic foot ulcers, and this coordination may be difficult to develop if conventional boundaries between healthcare providers are still in place. When the patient is cared for by independent teams of professional caregivers, the frequent co-occurrence of social and medical issues complicates supervision. When making management decisions, it is critical to consider the patient's (or his or her family's) needs and preferences, and the patient should play an important role in the process by making well-informed decisions. Every step of the way, patients and caregivers should receive advice from qualified health care professionals and should have easy access to a second opinion [36].

Conflict of interest

There is no conflict of interest among the authors.

Author details

Deephikaa Ramakrishnan Ramesh[1], Faiz Ahmed Shaikh[1*]
and Muhammad Ilyas Nadeem[2]

1 School of Pharmacy, Management and Science University, Shah Alam, Selangor, Malaysia

2 Faculty of Health and Life Sciences, Department of Healthcare Professional, Management and Science University, Shah Alam, Selangor, Malaysia

*Address all correspondence to: faizahmedskh@gmail.com

References

[1] Atlas D, Federation I. IDF. Brussels, Belgium: International Diabetes Federation; 2017. p. 2013

[2] Singh R, Kishore L, Kaur N. Diabetic peripheral neuropathy: Current perspective and future directions. Pharmacological Research. 2014;**80**:21-35

[3] Faruque LI, Wiebe N, Ehteshami-Afshar A, Liu Y, Dianati-Maleki N, Hemmelgarn BR, et al. Effect of telemedicine on glycated hemoglobin in diabetes: A systematic review and meta-analysis of randomized trials. CMAJ. 2017;**189**(9):E341-EE64

[4] Egan AM, Dinneen SF. What is diabetes? Medicine. 2019;**47**(1):1-4

[5] Roglic G. Global Report on Diabetes. World Health Organization. p. 86

[6] Khanolkar MP, Bain SC, Stephens JW. The diabetic foot. QJM. 2008;**101**:685-695

[7] Alavi A, Sibbald RG, Mayer D, Goodman L, Botros M, Armstrong DG, et al. Diabetic foot ulcers: Part I. Pathophysiology and prevention. Journal of the American Academy of Dermatology. 2014;**70**(1):1.e1-1.e18

[8] Wang A, Xu Z, Mu Y, Ji L. Clinical characteristics and medical costs in patients with diabetic amputation and nondiabetic patients with nonacute amputation in central urban hospitals in China. International Journal of Lower Extremity Wounds. 2014;**13**(1):17-21

[9] Muhammad-Lutfi A, Zaraihah M, Anuar-Ramdhan I. Knowledge and practice of diabetic foot Care in an in-patient setting at a tertiary medical center. Malaysian Orthopaedic Journal. 2014;**8**(3):22-26

[10] Bowering CK. Diabetic foot ulcers. Pathophysiology, assessment, and therapy. Canadian Family Physician. 2001;**47**:1-10

[11] Pendsey SP. Understanding diabetic foot. International Journal of Diabetes in Developing Countries. 2010;**30**(2):75. Available from: /pmc/articles/PMC2878694/

[12] Bakker K, Apelqvist J, Schaper NC. Practical guidelines on the management and prevention of the diabetic foot. Diabetes/Metabolism Research and Reviews. 2011;**28, 2012**:225-231

[13] IOP Conference Series: Earth and Environmental Science Pathophysiology Diabetic Foot Ulcer

[14] IDF Diabetes Atlas Seventh Edition 2015 by International Diabetes Federation—Issuu [Internet]. 2022. Available from: https://issuu.com/int._diabetes_federation/docs/idf_atlas_2015_uk/13

[15] Lim JZM, Ng NSL, Thomas C. Prevention and treatment of diabetic foot ulcers. Journal of the Royal Society of Medicine. 2017;**110**:104-109

[16] Pérez-Panero AJ, Ruiz-Muñoz M, Cuesta-Vargas AI, Gónzalez-Sánchez M. Prevention, assessment, diagnosis and management of diabetic foot based on clinical practice guidelines: A systematic review. Medicine. 2019;**98**(35):e16877. Available from: /pmc/articles/PMC6736276/

[17] Motley TA, Gilligan AM, Lange DL, Waycaster CR, Dickerson JE. Cost-effectiveness of clostridial collagenase ointment on wound closure in patients with diabetic foot ulcers: Economic

analysis of results from a multicenter, randomized, open-label trial. Journal of Foot and Ankle Research. 2015;**8**(1):1-12. DOI: 10.1186/s13047-015-0065-x

[18] Rosyid FN. Etiology, pathophysiology, diagnosis and management of diabetics' foot ulcer. International Journal of Research in Medical Sciences. 2017;**5**(10):4206

[19] Cardinal M, Eisenbud DE, Armstrong DG, Zelen C, Driver V, Attinger C, et al. Serial surgical debridement: A retrospective study on clinical outcomes in chronic lower extremity wounds. Wound Repair and Regeneration. 2009;**17**(3):306-311. DOI: 10.1111/j.1524-475X.2009.00485.x

[20] Edwards J, Stapley S. Debridement of diabetic foot ulcers. Cochrane Database of Systematic Reviews. 2010;(1). DOI: 10.1002/14651858.CD003556.pub2/full

[21] Diagnosis and Treatment of Diabetic Foot Infections on JSTOR [Internet]. 2022. Available from: https://www.jstor.org/stable/4462822

[22] Snyder RJ, Hanft JR. Diabetic foot ulcers—Effects on QOL, costs, and mortality and the role of standard wound care and advanced-care therapies. Ostomy/Wound Management. 2009;**55**(11):28-38. Available from: https://europepmc.org/article/med/19934461

[23] Alexiadou K, Doupis J. Management of diabetic foot ulcers. Diabetes Therapy. 2012;**3**(1):1-15. DOI: 10.1007/s13300-012-0004-9

[24] Watkins PJ. ABC of diabetes: The diabetic foot. British Medical Journal. 2003;**326**:977-979

[25] Kasiya MM et al. The challenge of diabetic foot care: Review of the literature and experience at Queen Elizabeth Central Hospital in Blantyre, Malawi. Malawi Medical Journal. 2017;**29**:218-223

[26] Overview: Diabetic Foot Problems: Prevention and Management: Guidance [Internet]. NICE. Available from: https://www.nice.org.uk/guidance/ng19 [Cited: 13 October 2022]

[27] Elias B, Chahine PD. Diabetic foot infections: An update on treatment [Internet]. U.S. Pharmacist – The Leading Journal in Pharmacy. 2013. Available from: https://www.uspharmacist.com/article/diabetic-foot-infections-an-update-on-treatment [Cited: 13 October 2022]

[28] Secretariat MA. Negative pressure wound therapy: An evidence-based analysis. Ont Health Technol Assess Ser. 2006;**6**(14):1. Available from: /pmc/articles/PMC3379164/

[29] Buchberger B, Follmann M, Freyer D, Huppertz H, Ehm A, Wasem J. The evidence for the use of growth factors and active skin substitutes for the treatment of non-infected diabetic foot ulcers (DFU): A health technology assessment (HTA). Experimental and Clinical Endocrinology and Diabetes. 2011;**119**(8):472-479. DOI: 10.1055/s-0031-1279713

[30] Hasan R, Firwana B, Elraiyah T, Domecq JP, Prutsky G, Nabhan M, et al. A systematic review and meta-analysis of glycemic control for the prevention of diabetic foot syndrome. Journal of Vascular Surgery. 2016;**63**(2):22S-28S.e2

[31] Diabetes [Internet]. MCR FEET. Available from: http://manchesterfeet.uk/diabetes/ [Cited: 13 October 2022]

[32] Callaghan BC, Little AA, Feldman EL, Hughes RA. Enhanced glucose control for preventing and

treating diabetic neuropathy. Cochrane Database of Systematic Reviews. 2012;(6). DOI: 10.1002/14651858. CD007543.pub2/full

[33] Bus SA, van Deursen RW, Armstrong DG, Lewis JEA, Caravaggi CF, Cavanagh PR. Footwear and offloading interventions to prevent and heal foot ulcers and reduce plantar pressure in patients with diabetes: A systematic review. Diabetes/Metabolism Research and Reviews. 2016;**32**:99-118. DOI: 10.1002/dmrr.2702

[34] Diabetic Foot Ulcer

[35] van Netten JJ, Price PE, Lavery LA, Monteiro-Soares M, Rasmussen A, Jubiz Y, et al. Prevention of foot ulcers in the at-risk patient with diabetes: A systematic review. Diabetes/Metabolism Research and Reviews. 2016;**32**:84-98. DOI: 10.1002/dmrr.2701

[36] van Houtum WH, Lavery LA. Regional variation in the incidence of diabetes-related amputations in the Netherlands. Diabetes Research and Clinical Practice. 1996;**31**(1-3):125-132

Section 3

Assessment

Chapter 8

Detection of Diabetic Foot Using Statistical Features

Saminathan Jayapal, Nandu Bhavani Murugesan and Sasikala Mohan

Abstract

Diabetes is a serious threat to universal health that respects neither socioeconomic rank nor nationwide boundaries. Diabetic foot and lower extremities problems, which affect 40 to 60 million people with diabetes universally, are a significant source of morbidity in people with diabetes. Conducting regular screening and risk stratification for at-risk feet can be greatly used for the management of blood glucose levels. Recent studies revealed that qualitative evidence can be attained using temperature variations from the thermogram of the plantar foot. The changes in temperature distribution are vital in the investigation of diabetic foot, which assist in the early detection of foot ulceration. The main objective of this work is to perform statistical analysis of diabetic foot to draw reasonable and accurate inferences. Besides, there is no gold standard method in classifying the plantar thermal images into any particular group. This may be conquered by quantitatively analyzing the temperature distributions in each foot separately. Since, plantar thermal images are colored in nature, certain color statistical features which are statistically more significant are added with the quantitative temperature distribution to develop an efficient machine learning method to prognosticate the likelihood of diabetes in patients with maximum accuracy is explored.

Keywords: diabetic foot, statistical analysis, Thermogram, machine learning, kernel mixer model

1. Introduction

Globally, diabetes is among the top ten causes of death in adults and was estimated to have caused the 4.2 million deaths resulting from diabetes and its complications in 2019. India is ranked second with almost 77 million cases in the list of countries that are most affected with diabetes while China leads the list with over 116.4 million diabetics. An estimated 15.8% (20.4 million) of live births are affected by hyperglycemia in pregnancy in 2019. This represents 9.3% of the world's population in this age group. In the International Diabetes Federation (IDF) South-East Asia Region, 57% of adults aged 20–79 years with diabetes are undiagnosed. An estimated 1.1 million children and adolescents (aged under 20 years) have type 1 diabetes. The total number is projected to rise to 578 million (10.2%) by 2030 and to 700 million (10.9%) by 2045.

Annual worldwide health spending on diabetes is estimated to be USD 760 billion. It is projected that expenditure will reach USD 825 billion by 2030 and USD 845 billion by 2045 [1].

Fifty percentage of patients with diabetes have some degree of neuropathy, resulting in at least one-foot ulcer throughout the lifetime in 15% of the cases. Neuropathic foot ulceration is a foremost cause of illness in patients with diabetes [2]. Diabetes patients have demonstrated that there are significantly increased skin temperatures and recognizable thermal radiation patterns, which differentiate them from healthy people. Thermometry of the diabetic foot is an impressive way to evaluate the risks associated with foot ulceration [3]. It has been revealed that monitoring foot skin temperature contributes to the clinical information before other medical signs of the wound can be recognized [4]. Differences in plantar thermal patterns in normal controls and non-ulcer diabetic patients were studied using thermometry [5]. Though, it has not been abundantly clarified to what extent the individual inconsistency of the plantar thermal patterns shows different trends between healthy and diabetes patients. Thermal imaging technology is capable to measure insignificant temperature irregularities to oversee some physiological circumstances [6]. Understanding of the temperature profile of foot is quite important to evolve thermal imaging system for detection of diabetic foot.

1.1 Temperature profile of foot

A healthy foot having healthy blood flow through healthy blood vessels whereas the decreased blood flow in the diabetic foot cause damage to organs like the leg and foot. The lack of blood flow caused by diabetes decreases the body's ability to heal from injuries. The assessment of raised temperature distribution with infrared thermometry in the diabetic foot is employed to identify the varying metabolic activity. Skin examination with an IR thermometer is flexible to repetitive wound care practice and home health. Nevertheless, the IR thermometry method becomes difficult and insufficient when measuring the temperature at many points on the foot [7, 8]. The liquid crystal thermograph methodology provides the temperatures pattern of the foot area as a colored foot imprint on a plate encompassed by layers of compressed thermochromics liquid crystals. The imprint persists for few minutes and then gradually disappear away. A temperature profile cannot be obtained for non-contact areas like an arch [9, 10].

Employing high-resolution and very sensitive thermal imaging cameras, the heat radiation from the matter is acquired and processed into an image of the thermal map which can then be stored and analyzed on screen and computer. Increased temperature investigation can be attained even for non-contact foot areas. Thermal images of diabetic feet reveal that it is 2.2°C colder than the lower leg, and usually the toes are not observable to the camera as they have become so hypothermic. Diabetic foot can arise several years before repetitive blood glucose levels indicate diabetes, and as such, can provide the patient time to treat the illness before everlasting nerve impairment occurs to the foot [11–13].

Though thermal imaging system is a promising screening tool for diabetic foot, diagnosis is usually done manually by skilled professionals. Hence, analyses made from thermograms are greatly subjective in nature. In order to overcome issues such as lack of proficient personnel, an efficient machine learning framework needs to be developed. The developments made in thermography and pattern recognition techniques are used to develop a competent system for detection of diabetic foot in plantar thermograms. Such a system can be used for screening of diabetes mellitus patients in developing countries, specifically by primary health care specialists in rural areas where health care expert is lacking.

2. Outline of the chapter

The main objective of this work is to perform statistical analysis in the thermal images to achieve reasonable and accurate inferences to make decisions accurately which aids in the prevention of numerous errors and biases. A Kernel Mixture Model (KMM) with four components approximates the plantar temperature distributions of the control group and DM group. Color texture features are extracted and analyzed to find the important features. A competent classification model to investigate the likelihood of diabetes in patients with maximum accuracy using the statistically significant temperature and color texture features is presented in **Figure 1**.

2.1 Thermal camera and dataset details

The camera specifications, dataset details, and image acquisition protocol used in this study are presented in the following sections.

2.1.1 Thermal camera specifications

Most of the work in plantar foot thermography has been done on thermograms acquired using an infrared thermal imaging camera. Thermal imaging cameras with a high resolution made suitable for medical applications can measure subtle temperature changes and hence are capable of improved detection of diabetic foot complications. A FLIR E60 thermal imaging camera is used for the present study to acquire plantar foot thermal images. It has a resolution of 320x240 pixels and covers a Field of View (FOV) of 25°x19°. The range of operation of the camera is in the region of the infrared spectrum from 7.5 μm to 13 μm wavelength. It can detect the temperature in the range of −20–650°C with thermal sensitivity of less than 0.05°C at 30°C and has an onboard digital camera with a resolution of 3.1 megapixels (MP). The onboard digital camera covers the same FOV as that of the thermal imaging camera and acquired images are of size 2048x1536 pixels. The temperature values are associated with a color palette (Rainbow Color Scheme palette) to represent and distinguish them graphically, where blue and green shades represent cooler regions. Warmer regions are represented by yellow, orange, and red colors in the increasing order of temperature respectively. Maximum temperature (intensity) is represented in white.

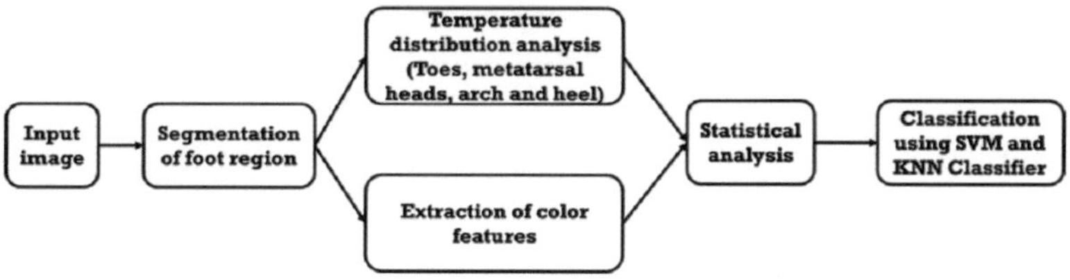

Figure 1.
Statistical analysis-based system for detection of diabetic foot.

It is ensured that the thermal imaging camera is calibrated against a black body reference as per the manufacturer's recommendations [14].

2.1.2 Laboratory and patient preparation protocols

In order to acquire accurate and convenient outcomes for clinical practice, the thermal images of the participants in the study were carried out in compliance with the protocols and guidelines set by the International Academy of Clinical Thermology Standards and Protocols [15–17] are listed below:

- The examination was performed in a steady-state 20 $\pm$ 1°C environment.
- The thermal images were acquired when the subject is sitting in a podiatric chair or comfortable and adequate position.
- The thermal imaging system emissivity is set to 0.98
- The thermal camera is calibrated prior to image acquisition by focusing lens on a black body
- After socks have been removed, the foot regions are cleaned with a damp towel
- All the subjects/patients are requested to remain in bare foot for 10–20 minutes before performing the actual measurements to eliminate the effect of external aspects on the temperature distributions of the foot
- The camera should be placed at a distance of 1.1 m
- During the investigation, the patient should be able to be placed relatively middle and sufficiently spaced from each wall
- Any IR radiation source is available in the investigational room that should be shielded/covered

The schematic representation of the acquisition of plantar thermal image is depicted in **Figure 2**.

2.1.3 Dataset details

The control subjects and Diabetes Mellitus (DM) patients were considered in this study. A total of 35 control subjects and 35 DM patients were recruited from and Hycare for Wounds, Chennai. Both control and DM groups comprise male and female participants, aged between 30 and 65 years. The DM group thermal image collection has been granted by Hycare for Wounds – Institutional Review Board. The participants were informed about the study beforehand and written informed consent forms were obtained from the participants of the study. Sample color and thermal images of the control group and DM group are acquired by the highly sensitive FLIR E60 IR thermal imaging system and are shown in **Figures 3** and **4** (a, b) respectively.

This study is carried out both on acquired and publicly available plantar thermogram database [17–21] for the early detection of diabetic foot. The plantar

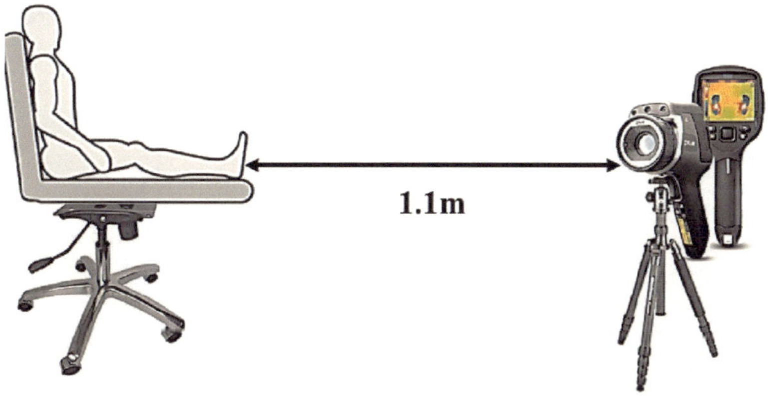

Figure 2.
Schematic arrangement for acquisition of thermal image.

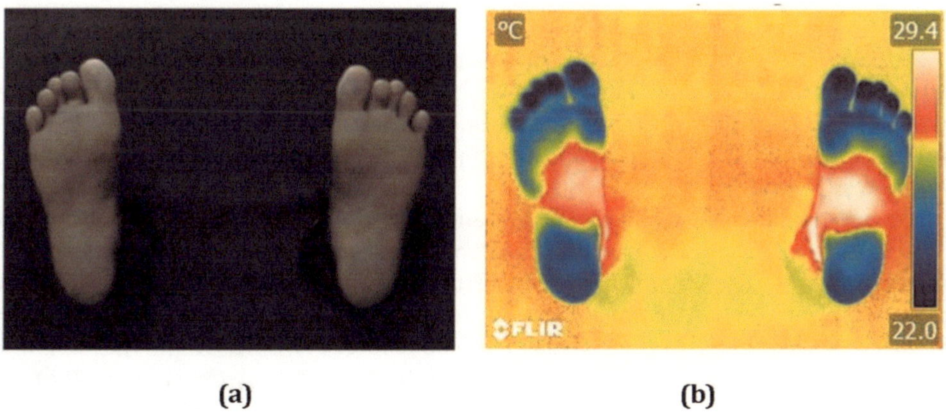

Figure 3.
Control group samples images. (a) Color image of the foot. (b) Thermal image of the foot.

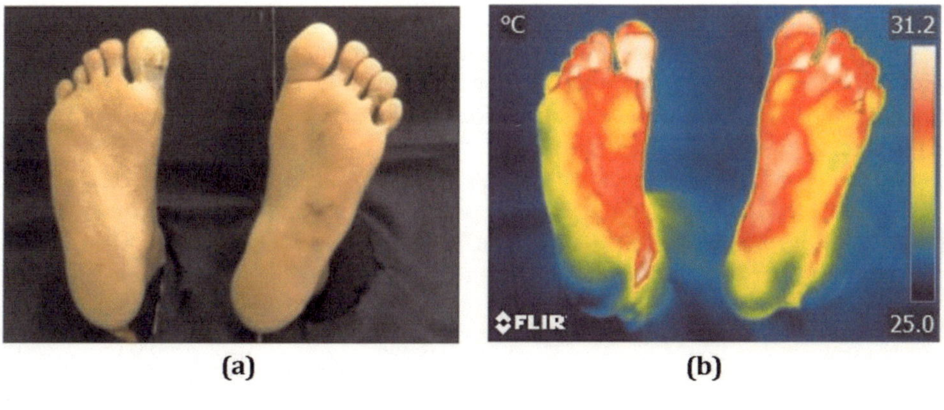

Figure 4.
DM group samples images. (a) Color image of the foot. (b) Thermal image of the foot.

thermogram database was obtained in a controlled environment 20 ± 1°C using FLIR E60 and FLIR E6 IR thermal imaging system from 122 subjects diagnosed with diabetes (DM group) and 45 healthy subjects (control group). During the thermogram

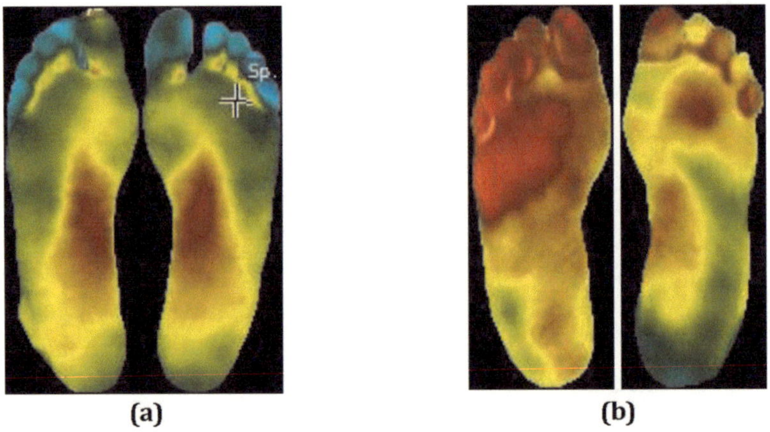

Figure 5.
(a) Database thermal image of the foot – Control group. (b) Database thermal image of the foot – DM group.

acquisition, the position of the camera is fixed by an adjustable vertical tripod to avoid any undesirable movement. The tripod is placed one meter away from the feet. The participants were asked to remove their shoes and socks and clean their feet with a damp towel. After that, the subjects were invited to maintain a supine position for 15 minutes (**Figure 5**).

For each plantar thermogram, the left and right foot were extracted and was taken as a separate thermogram, obtaining a database of 334 individual thermograms. The subjects were recruited from the General Hospital of the North, the General Hospital of the South, the BIOCARE clinic, and the National Institute of Astrophysics, Optics and Electronics (INAOE) over 3 years (from 2012 to 2014). The sample thermal image from the control group and DM group of the database is depicted in **Figure 4**(a) and (b), respectively. The total number of images used in the study is tabulated in **Table 1**, where the left foot and right foot is denoted by LF and RF respectively.

Since the database images are having only the foot region, the segmentation is performed only for the acquired plantar thermal images. The left and right foot regions are segmented from each color image using the region growing algorithm [22]. The red, green, and blue planes are extracted from thermal images and multiplied with the corresponding segmented foot region to get the ROI as a thermal image. The foot position of the left and right foot regions is corrected. **Figure 6**(a) and (b) show the segmented plantar foot regions of the control group and DM group, respectively. The raw temperature profiles of the acquired thermal images are exported as a.csv file from FLIR Tools® thermal analysis and reporting software. The binary image of the segmented foot regions is multiplied with the raw temperature profile of the corresponding foot regions to obtain the temperature distribution for the foot regions.

	Control Group	DM Group
Acquired images	70 (35 LF & 35 RF)	70 (35 LF & 35 RF)
Plantar thermogram database	90 (45 LF & 45 RF)	244 (122 LF & 122 RF)
Total	160 (80 LF & 80 RF)	314 (157 LF & 157 RF)

Table 1.
Number of images in the dataset.

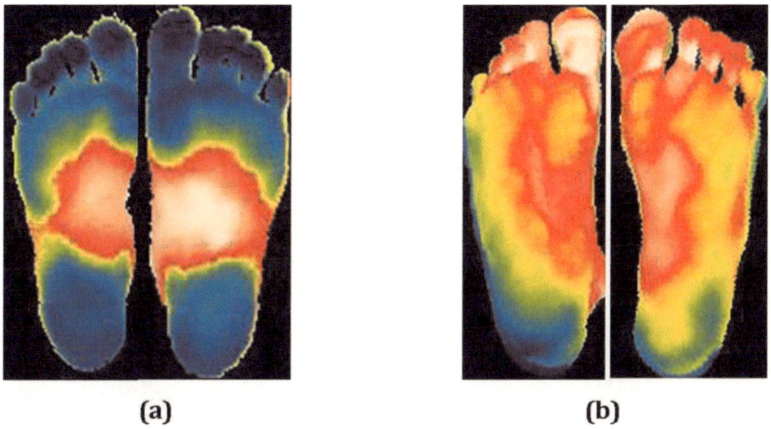

Figure 6.
(a) Segmented LF and RF regions of the control group. (b) Segmented left and right foot regions of the DM group.

3. Temperature distribution analysis

The plantar foot region is divided into four regions covering the toe region, metatarsal heads, medial arch and heel region to quantitatively analyze the temperature distribution. Histogram plot of the temperature distributions is accomplished by computing the mean temperature for each row of the plantar raw temperature profile for both left and right foot. The temperature values which are greater than 0°C are alone used to compute the mean temperature while those temperature values that are equal to 0°C are related to background and hence eliminated in each row. The histogram plot of the temperature distributions was offset corrected and normalized. The balance of every single distribution is eliminated by deducting the smallest temperature value either at the start or termination of the distribution. Later it is normalized by selecting a precision of three decimal figures to differentiate deviations in temperature from one pixel to another pixel.

3.1 Kernel density estimation

Once the final histogram is obtained, an approximation of density function is estimated using Kernel Density Estimation (KDE). A kernel distribution is a non-parametric representation of the probability density function (pdf) of a random variable. Let $x_1, x_2, \ldots, x_n$ be observations drawn independently from a distribution P with density p. The kernel density estimate $\hat{g}_h(x)$ is defined as

$$\hat{g}_h(x) = \frac{1}{nh}\sum_{i=1}^{n} K\left(\frac{x - x_i}{h}\right) \tag{1}$$

Where $K(\cdot)$ denotes the smoothing kernel function, and $h > 0$ is the smoothing bandwidth criterion which regulates the amount of smoothing. The kernel function is balanced and unimodal about the origin. The Gaussian kernel with normal distribution is utilized in this work. Bandwidth controls the smoothness of the density estimation. A smaller value of h will result in a rough estimation, while a higher value of h will result in a remarkably smooth estimate. The KDE smoothens every observation into a smaller density and the summation of these smaller densities together is used to attain the ultimate density estimate. The KDE is used to smooth the histogram plot of the temperature distribution and investigate the statistical significance [23, 24]. The temperature distributions of the four ROI (toes, metatarsal heads, medial arch and heel) in each foot are estimated using kernel density estimation. The histogram of the mean temperature distribution was smoothened using kernel density estimation which follows the non-parametric distribution. **Figures** 7 and **8** (a)-(d)

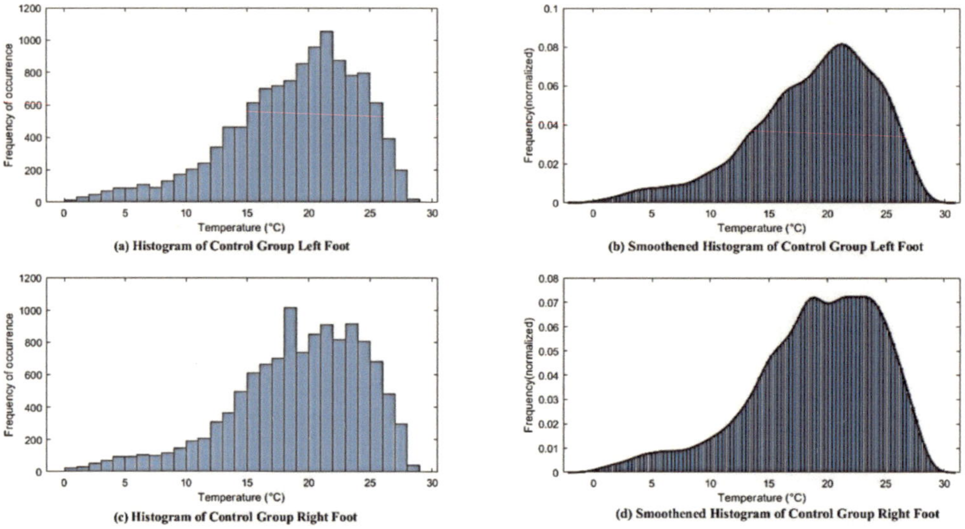

Figure 7.
Smoothened temperature distribution - control group.

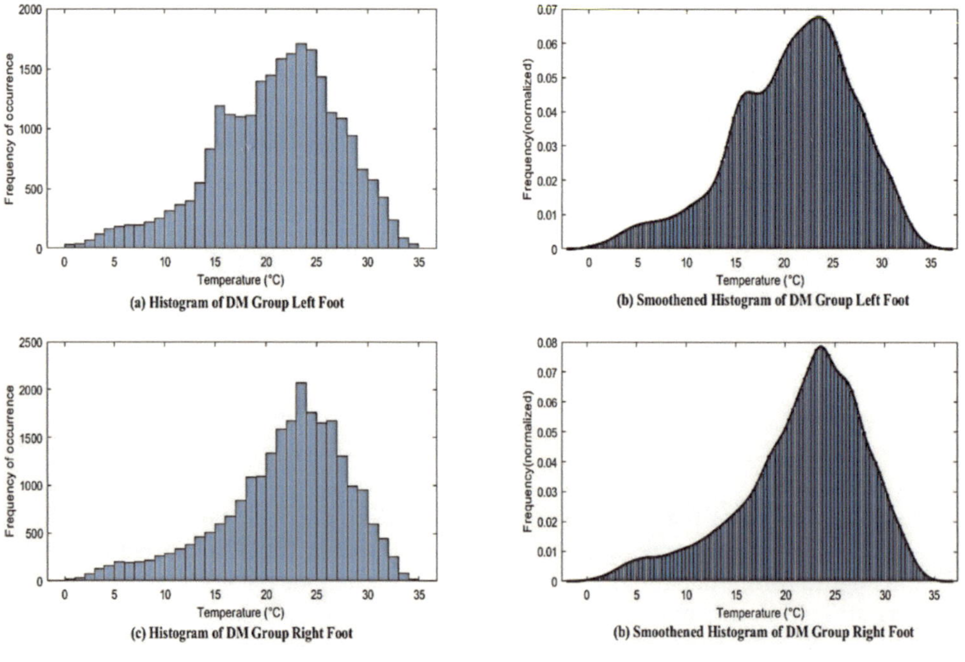

Figure 8.
Smoothened temperature distribution - DM group.

illustrates the histogram and smoothened histogram of the left and right foot for the control and DM group.

The smoothening is repeated for all the four regions of each left and right foot of the control and DM group. The region-wise smoothened temperature distribution is superimposed on the whole foot smoothened output for the control and DM groups depicted in **Figures 9** and **10**, respectively. From the mean temperature distribution histogram plot it was observed that the control group have a larger mean temperature around 21–22°C with a smaller number of occurrences of temperatures distribution while the DM group have a larger mean temperature around 23–24°C with a larger

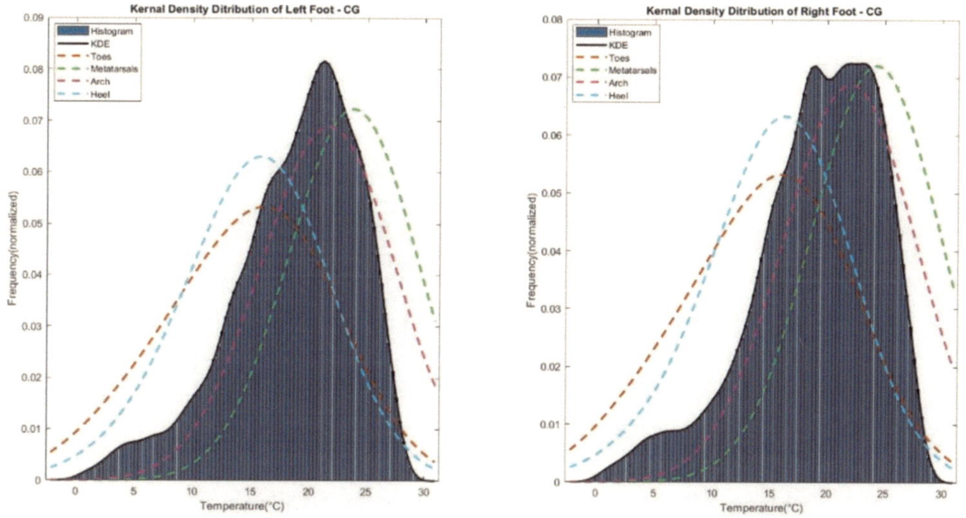

Figure 9.
Region wise smoothened temperature distribution superimposed on the whole foot - control group.

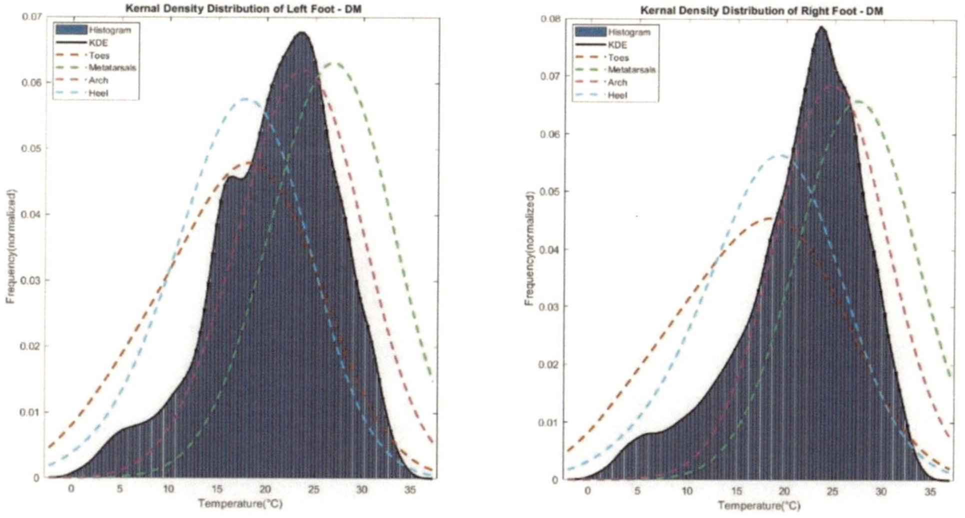

Figure 10.
Region wise smoothened temperature distribution superimposed on the whole foot output - DM group.

Group	Median (°C)		Interquartile Range (°C)	
	Left Foot	Right Foot	Left Foot	Right Foot
Control Group	27 ± 1.80	26.98 ± 1.77	1.92 ± 0.60	1.94 ± 0.49
DM Group	29.64 ± 2.85	29.84 ± 2.85	1.55 ± 0.66	1.59 ± 0.74

Table 2.
Median and interquartile range for whole foot.

Group	Region of Interest	Median (°C)		Interquartile Range (°C)	
		Left Foot	Right Foot	Left Foot	Right Foot
Control Group	Toes	25.3 ± 2.17	25.33 ± 2.32	1.68 ± 0.69	1.68 ± 0.64
	Metatarsals	26.9 ± 1.99	26.82 ± 1.93	1.00 ± 0.38	1.03 ± 0.35
	Arch	28.23 ± 1.63	28.19 ± 1.61	1.79 ± 0.56	1.82 ± 0.55
	Heel	26.69 ± 1.76	26.68 ± 1.75	1.19 ± 0.42	1.18 ± 0.41
DM Group	Toes	29.50 ± 3.66	29.72 ± 3.70	1.24 ± 0.79	1.32 ± 0.95
	Metatarsals	29.89 ± 3.15	30.12 ± 3.15	0.92 ± 0.52	0.89 ± 0.47
	Arch	29.86 ± 2.55	30.06 ± 2.52	1.24 ± 0.58	1.19 ± 0.56
	Heel	29.17 ± 2.73	29.45 ± 2.79	1.02 ± 0.42	1.08 ± 0.48

Table 3.
Region wise median and interquartile range.

number of occurrences of particular temperatures values. Similar kinds of deviations are observed in all the four ROIs of the left foot and right foot in the control and DM groups.

Since the KDE, which is a non-parametric distribution utilized to smoothen the temperature distribution, the central tendency among the control and DM groups was calculated by arranging the temperature distribution in ascending order to determine median and interquartile range for statistical analysis. Similarly, the median and interquartile range are also obtained for all the four ROIs with the corresponding smoothened temperature distribution for both control and DM groups. The computed median and interquartile range extracted from whole foot and region-wise for both groups are shown in **Tables 2** and **3**.

Thus, between **Tables 2** and **3** it was observed that the control group has a lower median temperature than the DM group. Since the mean temperature distribution is having a higher value in the lower quartile and upper quartile for the whole foot and region-wise, the interquartile range for the DM group is lesser than the control group.

The Chi-square goodness-of-fit [25] test was employed to assess the null hypothesis statistically for all the smoothened temperature distribution of left foot and right foot among control and DM group as shown in **Table 4**. This test is utilized to determine whether the variables are attained from the particular group temperature distribution or not and also to evaluate whether the sample data is representative of the full population of the temperature distribution. For both control and DM groups, the test returned an h value equivalent to one which specifies that chi-square goodness-of-fit rejects the null hypothesis at 5% significance level. Hence, these median and interquartile ranges are utilized to detect the diabetic foot in the classification process.

Group	Null Hypothesis (h)		Probability	
	Left Foot	Right Foot	Left Foot	Right Foot
Control Group	1	1	0.00459	0.00290
DM Group	1	1	0.00477	0.00448

Table 4.
Chi-square goodness-of-fit test results.

4. Extraction of color texture features

Color is one of the better notable and striking visual aspects that is employed in image retrieval and pattern recognition. Color moment (CM) is a computation technique utilized to discriminate images based on their color distribution in the image similar to the central tendency of the probability distribution. It is a potential technique for the description of color features [26, 27]. Once determined, these moments contribute a quantity for color resemblance among images. The red plane, green plane and blue plane images are extracted from each of the segmented thermal images for the control and DM groups. In this study, the mean (first moment), standard deviation (second moment), skewness (third moment), kurtosis (fourth moment), variance and entropy are extracted for all the four ROIs in each foot of all three color planes of images. The mean represents the average color value existing in the image. Variance is a measure of the color distribution of the image. Standard deviation is attained by executing a square root of the variance of the color distribution. Skewness is a measure of the degree of symmetry distribution of the color. The color textural features extracted from the green plane images of the left and right foot are highly correlated and shows very few dissimilarities within the values for all the four ROIs. Hence, the color texture features extracted from red and blue plane images alone are used for further processing. The skewness is having negative values for a few ROIs is the representation of the tail at the smaller end of the textural distribution is more pronounced than the tail at the larger end of the textural distribution.

5. Classification using machine learning techniques

5.1 Support vector machine

Support Vector Machine (SVM) is a discriminative classifier algorithm, concerning the patterns represented by the subset $d_i = +1$ and the patterns represented by the subset $d_i = -1$ are linearly separable. The decision surface that is in the form of a hyperplane that does the separation is given as follows.

$$w^T x = \sum_i w_i x_i \tag{2}$$

$$w^T x + b = 0 \tag{3}$$

where x is an input vector, w is an adjustable weight vector, and b is bias. The point closest to the hyperplane is called the 'support vector'. The SVM classifier maximizes the margin of separation between the classes and minimizes the classification errors [28, 29]. The best hyperplane for SVM is the one with the largest margin between the two classes.

5.2 K-nearest neighbors (KNN) classifier

The KNN classifier is a non-parametric, non-linear, and simple method that is used to classify the features. In this algorithm, the classification of test data is executed by finding a majority vote of the known class, and the input data will attain the class that is most common among its k-nearest neighbors [30, 31]. It is obtained using a distance metric such as Euclidean distance between the training and test data set which is calculated by

$$D_e(x_1, x_2) = \sqrt{\sum_{i=1}^{n} (x_{1i} - x_{2i})^2} \tag{4}$$

where, $x_1 = (x_{11}, x_{12}, \dots, x_{1n})$ and $x_2 = (x_{21}, x_{22}, \dots, x_{2n})$.

The test data is assigned to a class based on closest k-datasets for training based on resemblance measures, subsequently, the majority vote of the case neighbors is determined to categorize the case [32, 33].

The textural color features, median temperature and interquartile range forms the feature sets for detection of the diabetic foot using SVM and KNN classifier. The different grouping of feature sets which are extracted from the control and DM group was investigated in this study as follows:

- **Group 1 (RBT)** contains 14 features as it is formed with the statistical measure of the median, interquartile range with color textural features extracted from red and blue plane images

- **Group 2 (RB)** consists of 12 features as it is formed with the color textural features extracted from red and blue plane images

- **Group 3 (RT)** contains 8 features as it is formed with the statistical measure of the median, interquartile range with color textural features extracted from red plane images

- **Group 4 (BT)** consists of 8 features as it is formed with the statistical measure of the median, interquartile range with color textural features extracted from blue plane images

In all the combination, 80% of features are used to train and the remaining 20% of features are used to test the performance of the classifier. In this study, the classification is carried out using the SVM classifier and K-Nearest Neighbors (KNN) classifier for automatic classification of the plantar thermal images into two classes. The performance evaluation metrics of SVM and KNN classifiers for the detection of diabetic foot are shown in **Figure 11**. It was realized that the SVM classifier has obtained a higher classification accuracy of 92.86%, a sensitivity of 96.55%, specificity of 84.62%, a precision of 93.33%, and an F1-score of 94.92% for Group 1 (RBT) features combination than other combinations of feature set.

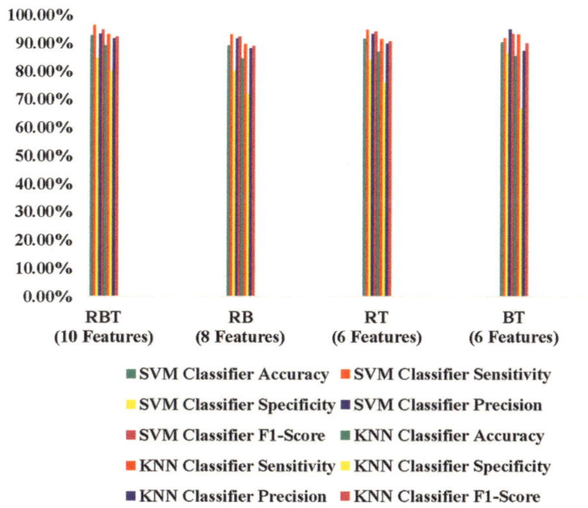

Figure 11.
Performance of SVM and KNN classifier in various combinations of feature set.

6. Conclusion

In this study, the statistical analysis of plantar temperature distribution based non-parametric way was done by using kernel density estimation. This approach showed the temperature distribution changes in different areas of the plantar region between the control and DM groups. The median and interquartile ranges are obtained from the statistical analysis. The extracted color features are grouped with the statistical measures of temperature distribution to automatically classify the data using SVM and KNN classifiers. Four different combinations of features sets were used to train and test the performance of the classifier. The SVM classier obtained better accuracy with Group 1 (RBT) feature sets.

Acknowledgements

Authors would like to register their profound gratitude to Dr.V.B. Narayanamurthy, Dr.K.Rajesh and Dr.R.Arvind, Directors of Hycare for Wouds, Chennai, India, for their help to get the ethical approval from Institutional Review Board (IRB) for acquisition of thermal images and Clinical inputs for the same. The authors are also thankful to the patients and healthy volunteers who actively participated in the data collection and the clinicians in the Hycare for Wounds, Chennai.

Conflict of interest

The authors declare no conflict of interest.

Author details

Saminathan Jayapal*, Nandu Bhavani Murugesan and Sasikala Mohan
Department of ECE, Anna University, College of Engineering, Guindy, Chennai, India

*Address all correspondence to: saminathan23@yahoo.in

References

[1] Diabetes Federation International, IDF Diabetes Atlas 2019. 2019. [Online]. Available: http://www.idf.org/about-diabetes/facts-figures

[2] Benbow SJ, Chan AW, Bowsher DR, Williams G, Macfarlane IA. The prediction of diabetic neuropathic plantar foot ulceration by liquid-crystal contact thermography. Diabetes Care. 1994;**17**(8):835-839

[3] Bharara M, Cobb JE, Claremont DJ. Thermography and thermometry in the assessment of diabetic neuropathic foot: A case for furthering the role of thermal techniques. International Journal of Lower Extremity Wounds. 2006;**5**(4): 250-260. DOI: 10.1177/15347346062 93481

[4] Armstrong DG, Holtz-Neiderer K, Wendel C, Mohler MJ, Kimbriel HR, Lavery LA. Skin temperature monitoring reduces the risk for diabetic foot ulceration in high-risk patients. The American Journal of Medicine. 2007; **120**(12):1042-1046. DOI: 10.1016/ j.amjmed.2007.06.028

[5] Nagase T, Sanada H, Takehara K, Oe M, Iizaka S, Ohashi Y, et al. Variations of plantar thermographic patterns in normal controls and non-ulcer diabetic patients: Novel classification using angiosome concept. Journal of Plastic, Reconstructive & Aesthetic Surgery. 2011;**64**(7):860-866. DOI: 10.1016/ j.bjps.2010.12.003 Epub 2011 Jan 22

[6] Mendes R, Sousa N, Almeida A, Vilaça-Alves J, Reis VM, Neves EB. Thermography: A technique for assessing the risk of developing diabetic foot disorders. Postgraduate Medical Journal. 2015;**91**(1079):538. BMJ Publishing Group. DOI: 10.1136/post gradmedj-2015-133441

[7] Sibbald RG, Mufti A, Armstrong DG. Infrared skin thermometry: an underutilized cost-effective tool for routine wound care practice and patient high-risk diabetic foot self-monitoring. Advances in skin & wound care. 2015; **28**(1):37-44; quiz 45-46. DOI: 10.1097/ 01.ASW.0000458991.58947.6b

[8] Ghosh A, Ray S, Garg MK, Chowdhury S, Mukhopadhyay S. The role of infrared dermal thermometry in the management of neuropathic diabetic foot ulcers. Diabetic Medicine. 2021;**38**(4):1-8. DOI: 10.1111/ dme.14368

[9] Stess RM, Sisney PC, Moss KM, Graf PM, Louie KS, Gooding GA, et al. Use of liquid crystal thermography in the evaluation of the diabetic foot. Diabetes Care. 1986;**9**(3):267-272

[10] Houghton VJ, Bower VM, Chant DC. Is an increase in skin temperature predictive of neuropathic foot ulceration in people with diabetes? A systematic review and meta-analysis. Journal of Foot Ankle Research. 2013;**6**(1):1-13. DOI: 10.1186/1757-1146-6-31

[11] Liu C, van der Heijden F, Klein ME, van Baal JG, Bus SA, van Netten JJ. Infrared dermal thermography on diabetic feet soles to predict ulcerations: A case study. Advanced Biomedical and Clinical Diagnostic Systems XI. 2013;**8572**:85720N. DOI: 10.1117/12. 2001807

[12] Bagavathiappan S, Saravanan T, Philip J, Jayakumar T, Raj B, Karunanithi R, et al. Investigation of peripheral vascular disorders using thermal imaging. The British Journal of Diabetes & Vascular Disease. 2008;**8**(2): 102-104. DOI: 10.1177/1474651408008 0020901

[13] Gatt A, Mercieca C, Borg A, Grech A, Camilleri L, Gatt C, et al. A comparison of thermographic characteristics of the hands and wrists of rheumatoid arthritis patients and healthy controls. Scientific Reports. 2019;**9**(1): 17204. DOI: 10.1038/s41598-019-53598-0

[14] Kirimtat A, Krejcar O, Selamat A, Herrera-Viedma E. FLIR vs SEEK thermal cameras in biomedicine: Comparative diagnosis through infrared thermography. BMC Bioinformatics. 2020;**21**(Suppl. 2):1-10. DOI: 10.1186/s12859-020-3355-7

[15] Picado ÁA, Elena EM, Beatriz GM. Standard protocol of preparation of the subject with risk foot for taking images by infrared thermography. Austin Endocrinology Diabetes Case Reports. 2018;**3**(1):1-5

[16] Hernandez-Contreras D, Peregrina-Barreto H, Rangel-Magdaleno J, Ramirez-Cortes J, Renero-Carrillo F. Automatic classification of thermal patterns in diabetic foot based on morphological pattern spectrum. Infrared Physics & Technology. 2015;**73**: 149-157. DOI: 10.1016/j.infrared.2015.09.022

[17] Hernandez-Contreras D, Peregrina-Barreto H, Rangel-Magdaleno J, Gonzalez-Bernal J. Narrative review: Diabetic foot and infrared thermography. Infrared Physics & Technology. 2016;**78**:105-117. DOI: 10.1016/j.infrared.2016.07.013

[18] Hernandez-Contreras D, Peregrina-Barreto H, Rangel-Magdaleno J, Carrillo FR. Plantar Thermogram database for the study of diabetic foot complications. IEEE Access. 2019. pp. 1-1. DOI: 10.1109/ACCESS.2019.2951356

[19] Hernandez-Contreras D, Peregrina-Barreto H, Rangel-Magdaleno J, Gonzalez-Bernal JA, Altamirano-Robles L. A quantitative index for classification of plantar thermal changes in the diabetic foot. Infrared Physics & Technology. 2017;**81**:242-249. DOI: 10.1016/j.infrared.2017.01.010

[20] Hernandez-Contreras D, Peregrina-Barreto H, Rangel-Magdaleno J, Ramirez-Cortes J, Renero-Carrillo F, Avina-Cervantes G. Evaluation of thermal patterns and distribution applied to the study of diabetic foot. IEEE. 2015;**2015**:482-487. DOI: 10.1109/I2MTC.2015.7151315

[21] Hernandez-Contreras D, Peregrina-Barreto H, and Rangel-Magdaleno J. Similarity measures to identify changes in plantar temperature distribution in diabetic subjects. In: 2018 IEEE International Autumn Meeting on Power, Electronics and Computing (ROPEC). 2018. pp. 1–6. DOI: 10.1109/ROPEC.2018.8661366

[22] Happ PN, Feitosa RQ, Bentes C, Farias R. A region-growing segmentation algorithm for GPUs. IEEE Geoscience and Remote Sensing Letters. 2013;**10**(6): 1612-1616. DOI: 10.1109/LGRS.2013.2272665

[23] Ledl T. Kernel Density Estimation: Theory and Application in Discriminant Analysis, Austrian Journal of Statistics. vol. 33, Issue no. 3, pp. 267–279, Apr. 2016

[24] Hang H, Feng Y, Suykens JA. Kernel density estimation for dynamical systems. Journal of Machine Learning Research. 2018;**19**:1-49

[25] van Netten JJ, van Baal JG, Bril A, Wissink M, Bus SA. An exploratory study on differences in cumulative

plantar tissue stress between healing and non-healing plantar neuropathic diabetic foot ulcers. Clinical biomechanics. 2018; **53**(2017):86-92. DOI: 10.1016/j.clinbiomech.2018.02.012

[26] Damayanti F, Muntasa A, Herawati S, Yusuf M, Rachmad A. Identification of Madura tobacco leaf disease using gray-level Co-occurrence matrix, color moments and Naïve Bayes. Journal of Physics: Conference Series. 2020;**1477**(5):1-8. DOI: 10.1088/1742-6596/1477/5/052054

[27] Jing J, Li Q, Li P, Zhang L. A new method of printed fabric image retrieval based on color moments and gist feature description. Textile Research Journal. 2016;**86**(11):1137-1150. DOI: 10.1177/0040517515606378

[28] Zhou Z, Yang J, Qi Y, Cai Y. Support vector machine and back propagation neutral network approaches for trip mode prediction using mobile phone data. IET Intelligent Transport Systems. 2018;**12**(10):1220-1226. DOI: 10.1049/iet-its.2018.5203

[29] Archibald R, Fann G. Feature selection and classification of hyperspectral images with support vector machines. IEEE Geoscience and Remote Sensing Letters. 2007;**4**(4):674-677. DOI: 10.1109/LGRS.2007.905116

[30] Mardini W et al. Enhanced detection of epileptic seizure using EEG signals in combination with machine learning classifiers. IEEE Access. 2020;**8**: 24046-24055

[31] Page A, Sagedy C, Smith E, Attaran N, Oates T, Mohsenin T. A flexible multichannel EEG feature extractor and classifier for seizure detection. IEEE Transactions on Circuits and Systems II: Express Briefs. 2015; **62**(2):109-113

[32] Eid MM, Yousef RN, Mohamed MA. A proposed automated system to classify diabetic foot from thermography. International Journal of Scientific and Engineering Research. 2018;**9**(12): 371-381

[33] Saadatfar H, Khosravi S, Joloudari JH, Mosavi A, Shamshirband S. A new k-nearest neighbors classifier for big data based on efficient data pruning. Mathematics. 2020;**8**(2):1-12. DOI: 10.3390/math8020286

Chapter 9

Assessment of Diabetic Foot

Manoharlal Manoj Abraham, Subramanian Hari Hara Sudan, Venugopal Pavithra, Nataraj Nithya, Pradhapsankar Veeramani and Suganya Murugeshan

Abstract

Diabetic Foot Complications are the main reason for hospitalization and amputation in people with diabetes. Globally ~435 million people have diabetes, with ~83–148 million of those estimated to develop foot ulcers in their lifetime. It is estimated that 16.8 million YLDs resulted from diabetic foot complications. Once an ulcer has developed, there is an increased risk of wound progression that may lead to amputation (~85% cases). In every 30 seconds, one lower limb amputation in diabetes patients occurs world-wide. The average cost for each amputation is over $70,000. American Podiatric Medical Association says that diabetic foot complications can be prevented by periodical Assessment of foot, which include visual inspection of bare foot; deformities, neurovascular abnormalities of foot and assessment of footwear. Relevant assessment and proactive foot care can reduce the burden of diabetic foot disease which will increase quality of life and reduce health care costs.

Keywords: diabetic foot ulcer, assessment, diabetic peripheral neuropathy, quality of life, prevention

1. Introduction

One of the most devastating consequences of diabetes mellitus is Diabetic Foot Disease (DFD) which represents a significant global burden for individuals and healthcare systems. It includes osseous degeneration, ulceration, and infection of the diabetic person's foot [1]. These are associated with neurologic abnormalities, various degrees of peripheral arterial disease, and metabolic complications of diabetes in the lower limb [2]. The signs of diabetic foot are changes in skin tone, skin temperature, swelling of the foot or ankle, discomfort in the legs, open blisters on the feet that are difficult to heal or are draining, corns or calluses, dry skin fissures, particularly around the heel, and odd or persistent foot odors are all symptoms to observe [3].

Diabetic foot symptoms vary from person to person and can depend on the particular problem the person is suffering at that moment. Symptoms include loss of sensation, numbness and tingling, blisters and other painless injuries, skin irritation and temperature changes, red streaks, injuries with or without discharge, painful tingling, and stains on socks. However, a person may also experience some of the following symptoms such as fever, feeling very sick, chills, uncontrollable blood sugar, shaking, shock, redness [4].

The first published diabetes-specific classification system, the Meggitt-Wagner system, is a simple system consisting of only six grades (0–5, 0 means intact skin), the first three is related to depth [5]. It's actually easy to use and may explain its popularity despite known limitations. For the sake of explanation, Peripheral Arterial Disease (PAD) and Infectious Diseases are not considered individually for superficial lesions and there is no mention of neuropathy. PAD is considered gangrene only at a later stage. Therefore, in clinical practice, the score is most often 2 or 3. This means that it is not accurate enough to isolate most lesions. Although its inaccuracies appear to be inadequate for research protocols, a systematic review of continuous wound healing by the International Working Group on Diabetic Foot shows that large works Meggitts - Wagner grade indicates the classification the patient population. Some other scales are used these are University of Texas wound classification system (UT), SAD system, the wound ischemia and foot infection classification (WIFI).

2. Pathophysiology

Diabetic peripheral neuropathy (loss of sensation) occurs typically 8–12 years after the onset of type 2 diabetes and is a tolerant factor for the development of ulcers. Diabetic peripheral neuropathy is a disorder of normal nerve activity throughout the body and can alter autonomic, motor, and sensory function [6]. Hyperglycemic conditions increase the production of several enzymes such as aldose reductase and sorbitol dehydrogenase. These enzymes convert glucose into sorbitol and fructose. The accumulation of these sugar products interferes with the synthesis of myo-inositol in nerve cells and impairs nerve conduction. In addition, hyperglycemic-induced microangiopathy results in reversible metabolic, motor and sensory nerve, immunological and ischemic damage leads to the autonomic nervous system dysfunction. It provokes low peripheral sensation and compensates for fine vasomotor control of pedal circulation and innervation of the small foot muscles. If the nerve is damaged, there is a risk of minor injuries, and when it is unnoticed an ulcer develops [7].

The microcirculation of the skin is controlled by the autonomic nervous system, when disturbed in Diabetes causes dryness and cracking of the skin, making it more susceptible to infections. These changes can help spread gangrene, ulcers, and loss of limbs [8, 9]. Hyperglycemia causes endothelial cell dysfunction, and smooth cell abnormalities in peripheral dysfunction include altered endothelial cell proliferation, basal membrane thickening, decreased nitrogen monoxide synthesis, increased blood density, altered microvascular tone, and blood flow. Clinically the case may have signs of vascular insufficiency such as claudication, night pain or rest pain, absent peripheral pulses, thinning of the skin, loss of limb hair, etc. [6].

3. Importance of assessment

Foot disease affects almost 6% of diabetics and is associated with infections, ulcers, or destruction of foot tissue. Most ulcers can be prevented with proper foot care and screening of foot risk factors at risk of complications [9–11]. Uncontrolled diabetes contributes to the development of neuropathy and peripheral arterial disease through complex metabolic pathways. Loss of sensation due to peripheral neuropathy, ischemia due to peripheral arterial disease, or a combination thereof can cause foot ulcers. Thorough foot examination is important for early detection of the disease. Screening for peripheral neuropathy and peripheral arterial disease helps identify patients at risk for foot ulcers. Assess the patient's general condition for signs of toxicity or sepsis, such as circulation or breathing, with or without malaise, poor appearance, abnormal behavior, and fever. At each follow-up schedule, examine feet for ulcers/gangrene. The purpose of screening is to identify patients who have lost foot protection [12, 13].

To identify diabetic patients at risk of ulcers, foot examinations are needed, including nervous and vascular system, skin disorders, and foot structure. According to age and length of diabetes, diabetic peripheral neuropathy, itself that affects up to 50% of diabetics and it is the most ubiquitous and crippling consequence of Diabetes mellitus. Peripheral senses (small and large nerve fibers) and motor nerves are affected by this condition, which is marked by significant axonal degeneration and segmental demyelination [14–16].

4. Neurological assessment of diabetic foot

The clinical assessment of diabetic foot ulcer is currently subjective and limited, hampering effective diagnosis, treatment and prevention. Population-based studies report that the annual incidence of foot ulcers in diabetics is estimated to have DFU throughout their lives [17–19]. Once onset, despite treatment, foot ulcers may take weeks or months to heal, or may not heal at all. In addition, DFU is repeated frequently. Approximately 40% of patients will relapse within 1 year and 60% of patients will relapse within 3 years. The DFU not only reduces an individual's quality of life, but also has significant economic and social implications in the form of increased hospitalization rates, cost of care, and reduced patient mobility [20].

Most guidelines recommend 10 g of monofilament to assess neuropathy in diabetic patients. This test can be combined with another test to screen for neuropathy. Biothesiometer or graduated tuning fork (Rydel Seiffer) to determine the vibration perception threshold [21, 22]. The Modified Neuropathy Disorder Score (NDS) tests (**Table 1**) different sensory modalities of the foot and ankle - (i) vibration perception (using a 128 Hz sound fork), (ii) temperature perception (warm/cold), (iii). Pain (sharp/dull) and (iv) ankle jerk reflex- score range is 0 to 10, 0 for intact sensation and 10 for complete numbness with DPN. The Vibration Perception Threshold (VPT) is a semi-quantitative measure of sensory perception, usually placed at the tip of the toe and measured with a neuro or biothesiometer. VPT displays 0–50 volt readings, where 50 volt indicates complete numbness of DPN. Severe DPNs are usually stratified by VPTs with a modified NDS score of 6 or higher (or) of 25 volts or higher [22–25].

Inadequate foot protection due to nerve injury (neuropathy) does not result in compensatory mechanisms for painful stimuli such as dragging/gait changes to redistribute foot pressure. Continued inflammation results in enzymatic autolysis with tissue destruction and ulcers. The main goal of DFU clinical practice is to prevent the formation of ulcers through early detection and intervention. This reflects the challenges and medical costs associated with effective treatment after the onset of an ulcer. Regular foot evaluation and training are recommended for people with diabetes. This process is usually stratified by the risk of developing an ulcer. Current risk assessments are clinical and subjective, assessing the presence of callus as a surrogate marker for neuropathy, foot malformations, and high sole load, and for medium-risk or high-risk individual therapeutic footwear is recommended [26, 27].

Clinical evaluation tools require special training of clinical examiners to make accurate assessments based on patient outcomes. This assessment helps to efficiently

Neuropathy Disability Score (NDS)			
		Right	**Left**
Vibration perception threshold 128 Hz tuning fork; apex of big toe; trial pair = vibrating, nonvibrating (hit the wrong end of the tuning fork); normal = can distinguish vibrating / not vibrating	Subject sitting, eyes closed, legs outstretched: demonstrate on clavicle or dorsum of hand; in each case repeat three pairs of trials (mix up stimulus order within trial pair, in each case maintain stimulus 2 seconds); in each case ask "do you feel vibration / cold / sharp now or now?"; abnormal is at least two of three trials wrong or "cannot tell" normal = 0 abnormal = 1		
Temperature perception Rest Tip-Therm rod on dorsum of foot, trial pair = plastic end ("not cold"), metal end ("cold"); normal = can distinguish cold / not cold			
Pin-prick Apply Neurotip on proximal big toe just enough to deform skin; trial pair = sharp end, blunt end; normal = can distinguish sharp / not sharp			
Achilles reflex Kneeling on a chair, upright holding back of chair; stretch tendon to ankle neutral first; reinforcement – hook fingers together and pull when asked	present = 0 present with reinforcement = 1 absent = 2		
NDS Total out of 10			

Table 1.
NDS.

identify patients at risk and monitor whether they need intervention. The Assessment should also be based on an assessment of diabetic foot ulcer and risk of amputation, healing of diabetic foot ulcer, and assessment of diabetic foot ulcer infection [28]. Outcome measures for assessing diabetic neuropathy such as Utah Early Neuropathy Scale (UNES), for Ulcer risk (Queensland high-risk foot form or QHRFF); Diabetic foot ulcer assessment, scoring and amputation risk (Perfusion, Extent, Depth, Infection and Sensory scale or PEDIS); Site, Ischemia, Neuropathy, Bacterial infection and Depth assessment (SINBAD); Diabetic foot ulcer measurement (Leg Ulcer Measurement Tool LUMT) have been shown to be effective and valid.

An advanced home assessment tool for monitoring the feet of diabetics is desirable, and measuring the skin temperature of these feet is a promising modality. Temperature assessment is based on the idea that skin heat as a predictor of diabetic foot ulcer [29].

5. Vascular assessment of diabetic foot

Anatomical arterial disease can result in a more severe kind of perfusion deficit in patients with Diabetes and it is due to the paucity of collateral vessels and also the influence of physiological factors like arteriolar shunting and neuropathy associated with Diabetes [30]. A complete physical examination should be carried out in any patient with Diabetic foot ulceration, particularly, a detailed medical history and assessment of peripheral pulses – however, clinical examination alone cannot reliably assess the severity of perfusion deficit [31]. In order to perform a detailed assessment of the peripheral artery and its perfusion, more tests are indeed necessary.

Commonly used imaging techniques like Duplex ultrasound and Angiography allow only the assessment of the morphological distribution of Peripheral artery disease and also provide some information on the global perfusion deficit. Patients with Ischaemic foot ulceration have compartmental perfusion deficit, in which the degree of perfusion at the actual area of tissue loss cannot be identified. Therefore, assessment of foot perfusion in a patient with diabetic foot ulcer should also include the regional tissue perfusion deficit [30].

5.1 Assessment of disease severity

The patients with diabetic foot ulceration should be evaluated for the presence of Peripheral artery disease during the time of presentation and they have to be managed in a multi-disciplinary setting [32–34]. The assessment of disease severity can be carried out using Ankle brachial pressure index, Toe pressures and Pulse volume recordings.

5.1.1 Ankle brachial pressure index

Doppler measure Ankle brachial pressure index is most commonly used to screen the presence of Peripheral artery disease. However, Ankle brachial pressure index and other routinely performed non – invasive bedside tests otherwise useful in the assessment of Peripheral artery disease may be unreliable in patients with Diabetes [35]. Ankle brachial pressure index score of <0.9 is indicative of impaired blood flow; however the finding of a normal Ankle brachial pressure index in a person with diabetes is not reliable – increased arterial stiffness may reduce distal flow [36] and medial arterial calcification, resulting in incompressible vessels which may in turn causes falsely elevated pressures.

5.1.2 Toe pressures

Toe pressure and toe arm pressure index (TBI) may be a more useful measure of perfusion due to the characteristic sparing of the foot arteries from vascular disease in diabetics [30]. Toe pressure can be effectively measured using photoplethysmography (which detects pulsating flow to generate pulse wave waveforms) or laser Doppler (which detects wavelength changes when a laser hits blood cells).

5.1.3 Pulse volume recordings

Pulse rate records are also used to identify the presence of arterial disease. The amount of pulse wave corresponds to the cardiac cycle-rapid upstrokes and sharp spikes occur during systole, gradually slopes down during diastole, followed by reflective waves (dicrotic notches). In the presence of arterial disease, the waveform flattens and the pulse width widens. When pulse volume recordings are used in lower limbs, the changes in the waveform denotes the general location of significant disease, whereas it assesses the total blood flow through the area and cannot give accurate information regarding the exact location of the disease [30]. Pulse volume recordings are useful in patients with Diabetes who have falsely elevated Ankle brachial pressure index because of calcified vessels [37], as the effect of calcification on the waveform is usually distinguishable from that because of obstructive arterial disease.

5.2 Assessment of morphological distribution

The anatomical distribution of the disease in patients with diabetic foot ulcer is to determine if revascularization is necessary and, if necessary, which method (intra-vascular or open surgery) is appropriate and useful. The main challenge in imaging the arterial tree of diabetics is the characteristically complex anatomical distribution of the disease [30].

5.2.1 Duplex ultrasound

Color duplex ultrasound is the first imaging technique used to examine patients with peripheral arterial disease. The patients with Diabetes have a diffuse and distal arterial disease; detailed imaging studies along with duplex ultrasound need to be used for pre – operative investigation while planning for revascularization.

5.2.2 Angiography

Detailed morphological information can be provided by Angiography. Traditional digital subtraction angiography (DSA) is the gold standard method cannot fully identify patent distal vessels for which Magnetic resonance angiography (MRA) can be used [30].

5.3 Assessment of regional tissue perfusion

Assessment of local tissue perfusion is more useful in understanding the perfusion deficit at the exact area and also helps to estimate the healing tendency. Diabetic patients need this assessment, as global perfusion assessment measures usually do not reflect the regional deficit, due to poor collateralization found in them.

5.3.1 Transcutaneous oxygen tension (Tcpo$_2$)

Transcutaneous oxygen tension (TcPO$_2$) measurement is an established method of evaluating the cutaneous perfusion and it is also more sensitive in detecting Peripheral artery disease than Ankle brachial pressure index in patients with Diabetes [38]. TcPO$_2$ measures the transfer of oxygen molecules to the skin surface and a reduction in transcutaneous oxygen tension is commonly in patients with Peripheral artery disease [39]. TcPO$_2$ values may be paradoxically increased in patients with Diabetes due to arteriolar shunting in the microcirculation and is also affected by the metabolic demands of the tissue being assessed.

5.3.2 Skin perfusion pressure

Skin perfusion pressure has been used as a successful measure to assess the lower limb ischaemia severity and also analyses the chances of wound healing and thereby helps in selecting the appropriate level of amputation [40, 41].

5.3.3 Fluorescence angiography

It commonly uses Indocyanine green dye (ICG) for measuring the fluorescence intensity at various areas of the involved limb, thereby allows a semi – quantitative measurement of regional perfusion and identifies the superficial collaterals in patients with arterial occlusions [30]. It is also used in patients with critical limb ischaemia to provide more rapid and quantitative information about foot perfusion [42].

5.3.4 Laser Doppler techniques

Laser Doppler flowmetry is used to measure the local microcirculatory blood perfusion by using a beam of Laser light which is partially absorbed when it hits the tissue being evaluated, to a depth of up to 1 mm. The change in wavelength like magnitude and frequency can be converted into a measurement thereby representing the relative perfusion than absolute values. It has been used to identify poor perfusion in lower extremity ulcers [43].

Hence a comprehensive assessment of foot perfusion in Diabetes patients should therefore include anatomical assessments of structural arterial disease combined with evaluation of regional tissue perfusion. The most commonly available techniques also have certain limitations while relating to the complexity of Diabetes. Novel techniques which are meant to assess muscle and deep tissue perfusion are under the process of development, which are more likely to be used widely in the near future.

6. Biomechanical assessment of diabetic foot

Peripheral neuropathy causes changes in foot function as well as in structure (due to prominent Metatarsal heads), dryness of the skin which in turn can end up in excessive callus formation [44–46]. An important risk factor for the development of Diabetic foot ulceration is high plantar foot pressure [47, 48]. In patients with Diabetes, limited joint mobility in the ankle and foot complex also had suggested to increase plantar pressure [49, 50] and also to be related with foot ulceration [51, 52]. The prevalence of limited joint mobility varies between 49% and 58% in Type I Diabetes patients and between 45% and 52% in Type II Diabetes patients [53, 54].

Most of the Diabetic foot ulcers occur in the forefoot, mainly under the metatarsal heads and under the digits (hallux). When the metatarsal head makes contact with the ground, it usually contacts at a single point because the inferior aspect of each metatarsal head is usually round.

The main structure responsible for dissipating the pressure from the lowest point of the metatarsal heads, to the sides of the metatarsal heads, then to the intermetatarsal spaces and to the points which are proximal and distal to the metatarsal heads is Metatarsal fat pad [55]. Patients with diabetes with or without neuropathy generally have decreased thickness in the metatarsal fat pads. The thinner the metatarsal fat pad, the higher the risk of developing Diabetic foot ulcers [56, 57]. The easiest way to measure fat pad thickness under the metatarsal heads is by using Ultrasound [58].

A softer metatarsal fat pad increases the shock absorption of the forefoot while hitting the ground, whereas a stiffer metatarsal fat pad decreases shock absorption thereby greater energy gets imparted to the soft tissues while landing on the forefoot [59]. The stiffer metatarsal fat pad prevents the load from being distributed medially and laterally from the deepest point of the metatarsal head. Therefore, more stress is applied to the soft tissue pad just below the metatarsophalangeal head, and less stress is applied to the part of the fat pad between the metatarsophalangeal heads [60].

In Diabetes, the collagen in the plantar fat pad not only stiffness but also the collagen tissues throughout the body stiffen. This stiffening of the entire collagen tissue causes all ligaments to become stiff and all joints to lose mobility [61]. Thus it can be a serious issue for most phase of the Gait cycle.

During the stance phase of gait, the hind foot begins with a slight inversion and then eversion. The forefoot first lands on the fifth metatarsal head, then each metatarsal lands from lateral to medial. At the end of the stance phase, the hind foot is slightly everted and the fore foot is slightly inverted. If a diabetic presents a normal amount of hind foot eversion during contact, the forefoot may be difficult to compensate by inverting at the mid tarsal joints. It can increase the pressure under the first and second metatarsal heads. On the other hand, if the forefoot cannot be fully inverted to pronate the sub talar joint, the pressure under the 4th and 5th metatarsal heads will increase. Coronal and sagittal movements are also reduced in all metatarsals with stiffer collagen tissue [62].

The glycation of the Achilles tendon increases the tendon's thickness and stiffness [63, 64]. It in turn causes several changes in the diabetic foot, including earlier forefoot loading at contact as well as an increased load on the forefoot during the stance phase of gait [65, 66]. The thickening of plantar fascia happens along with the thickening of the Achilles tendon [67]. The thickened Achilles tendon decreases the effect of windlass mechanism of the foot, which further decreases the dorsiflexion of the digits, decreased time in the propulsive period of gait and a decrease in the supination of the hind foot during foot propulsion [68, 69]. Diabetic neuropathy has a greater adverse effect on the foot. Tissue glycation is the predicting factor of other diabetic complications including neuropathy. The joint mobility of the subtalar joint is significantly reduced in the ulcerated foot than the contra lateral non ulcerated foot in Diabetic neuropathic patients [47]. Hence, combination of neuropathy and trauma results in breakdown of tissue. Increased plantar pressure can be contributed to the alterations in the foot shape, presence of callus and limited joint mobility.

Kinematic analysis was performed on the knees and ankles using 3D SIMI REALITY MOTION SYSTEM GmbH, Germany, two Basler high-speed cameras (1394a/b, GigE, 100fps @ 1Megapixel). We used Kinetik I-Step software (Aetrex, USA) and Wintrack Dynamic Scan Floor Mat (Medicapteure software, France, USA). Significant differences in kinematic and kinematic variables such as toe-off knee angle, static knee speed, heel strike, mid-stance and toe-off, static knee acceleration, heel strike and mid-stance, and ankle joint angle, Mid stance, static ankle speed, heel strike and mid stance, static ankle acceleration, heel strike, mid stance and toe off, walk cycle duration, maximum average sole pressure and maximum ankle pressure Was recognized. Therefore biomechanical analysis is an important tool and can be used for early screening and prediction of altered kinematic and kinetics in diabetes mellitus [70].

7. Conclusion

Patients may not receive the podiatry follow-up necessary to identify warning signs of recurrence and provide appropriate management. To guide preventive strategies, it is necessary to fully understand the factors that predict the recurrence of ulcers. The strongest predictor of diabetic foot ulcer is the previous foot ulcer. A study of patients with healed foot ulcers has shown that early signs of skin damage such as heavy calluses, blisters, and bleeding are one of the strongest predictors of ulcer recurrence. If these pre-ulcer lesions are recognized early, their treatment can probably prevent the recurrence of many ulcers [21].

Low-risk individuals may progress to medium-risk or high-risk and should continue their foot examinations annually. More frequent follow-up is recommended for medium-risk or high-risk patients. Patients with foot malformations or patients diagnosed with peripheral neuropathy or peripheral arterial disease at baseline. Introducing prophylactic foot care services for basic nail and skin care including, wound resection of callus, for patients with callus and deformed toe nail. Timely referrals to foot protection services to manage risk factors for diabetics prevent infection, gangrene, amputation, or death, reducing hospitalization and costs [22].

Acknowledgements

The authors sincerely thank Dr. G. Bakthavathsalam, Chairman, Mrs. Vasanthi Ragu, Vice Chairman, Mr. Prabhu Kumar, CEO, and Prof V. Mohan Gandhi, CEO, KG Hospital, Coimbatore, India, for their support.

Conflict of interest

The authors declare no conflict of interest.

Author details

Manoharlal Manoj Abraham*, Subramanian Hari Hara Sudan, Venugopal Pavithra, Nataraj Nithya, Pradhapsankar Veeramani and Suganya Murugeshan
K. G College of Physiotherapy (Affiliated to the Tamil Nadu Dr. M.G.R Medical University, Chennai), Coimbatore, India

*Address all correspondence to: abraham.physio@gmail.com

References

[1] Bowling FL, Foley KJ, Boulton AJM. Chapter 14 - Diabetic foot. In: Tavakoli M, editor. Diabetic Neuropathy. Elsevier. 2022. pp. 223-234. ISBN 9780128206690. Available from: https://doi.org/10.1016/B978-0-12-820669-0.00022-0

[2] Tiwari S, Pratyush DD, Dwivedi A, Gupta SK, Rai M, Singh SK. Microbiological and clinical characteristics of diabetic foot infections in northern India. Journal of Infection in Developing Countries. 2012;**6**:329-332

[3] Michael Dansinger. Diabetic Foot Problems. 2021. Available from: https://www.webmd.com/diabetes/foot-problems. [Accessed: July 2, 2022]

[4] Kelly Wood. How Can Diabetes Affect the Feet? 2022. Available from: https://www.medicalnewstoday.com/articles/317504. [Accessed: July 2, 2022]

[5] Game FL, Apelqvist J, Attinger, C, Hartemann A, Hinchliffe RJ, et al. and on behalf of the International Working Group on the Diabetic Foot (IWGDF) Effectiveness of interventions to enhance healing of chronic ulcers of the foot in diabetes: A systematic review. Diabetes/Metabolism Research and Reviews. 2016;**32**:154-168. DOI: 10.1002/dmrr.2707.

[6] Edition S. IDF diabetes atlas. International Diabetes Federation. 2015

[7] Singh S, Pai RP, Yuhhui C. Diabetic foot ulcer-diagnosis and management. Clinical Research Foot Ankle. 2013;**1**(3):1-9

[8] Armstrong DG, Boulton AJM, Bus SA. Diabetic foot ulcers and their recurrence. The New England Journal of Medicine. 2017;**376**:2367-2375

[9] Zhang P, Lu J, Jing Y, Tang S, Zhu D, Bi Y. Global epidemiology of diabetic foot ulceration: A systematic review and meta-analysis (†). Annals of Medicine. 2017;**49**:106-116. DOI: 10.1080/07853890.2016.1231932

[10] Schaper NC, Apelqvist J, Bakker K. The international consensus and practical guidelines on the management and prevention of the diabetic foot. Current Diabetes Reports. 2003;**3**:475-479. DOI: 10.1007/s11892-003-0010-4

[11] Singh N, Armstrong DG, Lipsky BA. Preventing foot ulcers in patients with diabetes. JAMA. 2005;**293**:217-228. DOI: 10.1001/jama.293.2.217

[12] Mishra SC, Chhatbar KC, Kashikar A, Mehndiratta A. Diabetic foot. BMJ. 2017:359

[13] Bhat S, Mary S, Giri AP, Kulkarni MJ. Advanced glycation end products (AGEs) in diabetic complications. In: Kartha CC, Ramachandran S, Pillai RM, editors. Mechanisms of Vascular Defects in Diabetes Mellitus. Series: Advances in biochemistry in health and disease (17). Springer: Cham; 2017; pp. 423-449. ISBN 9783319603230. DOI: 10.1007/978-3-319-60324-7_19

[14] Reeves ND, Orlando G, Brown SJ. Sensory-motor mechanisms increasing falls risk in diabetic peripheral neuropathy. Medicina. 2021;**57**(5):457

[15] Pop-Busui R, Boulton AJ, Feldman EL, Bril V, Freeman R, Malik RA, et al. Diabetic neuropathy: A position statement by the American Diabetes Association. Diabetes Care. 2017;**40**:136-154

[16] Said G. Diabetic neuropathy—A review. Nature Clinical Practice. Neurology. 2007;**3**:331-340

[17] Wang L, Jones D, Chapman GJ, Siddle HJ, Russell DA, Alazmani A, et al. A review of wearable sensor systems to monitor plantar loading in the assessment of diabetic foot ulcers. IEEE Transactions on Biomedical Engineering. 2019;**67**(7):1989 2001

[18] International Diabetes Federation. IDF Diabetes ATLAS Eighth Edition [Online]. 2017. Available: http://www.diabetesatlas.org/. [Accessed: September 10, 2018]

[19] G. Leese et al., "Stratification of foot ulcer risk in patients with diabetes: A population-based study," International Journal of Clinical Practice, vol. 60, no. 5, pp. 541-545, May 2006.

[20] Hoogeveen RC, Dorresteijn JA, Kriegsman DM, Valk GD. Complex interventions for preventing diabetic foot ulceration. The Cochrane database of systematic reviews. 2015;**8**:CD007610. Available from: https://doi. org/10.1002/14651858.CD007610.pub3

[21] International Guidelines Team. National Institute for Health and Care Excellence clinical guideline 19. Diabetic foot problems: prevention and management. 2016. www.nice.org.uk/guidance/ng19

[22] Bus SA, van Netten JJ, Lavery LA, et al. International working group on the diabetic foot guidance on the prevention of foot ulcers in at-risk patients with diabetes. Diabetes/Metabolism Research and Reviews. 2016;**32**:16-24. DOI: 10.1002/dmrr.2696

[23] Boulton AJ, Malik RA, Arezzo JC, Sosenko JM. Diabetic somatic neuropathies. Diabetes Care. 2004;**27**:1458-1486

[24] Almurdhi MM, Reeves ND, Bowling FL, Boulton AJM, Jeziorska M, Malik RA. Reduced lower-limb muscle strength and volume in patients with type 2 diabetes in relation to neuropathy, intramuscular fat, and vitamin D levels. Diabetes Care. 2016;**39**:441-447

[25] Almurdhi MM, Brown SJ, Bowling FL, Boulton AJM, Jeziorska M, Malik RA, et al. Altered walking strategy and increased unsteadiness in participants with impaired glucose tolerance and type 2 diabetes relates to small-fibre neuropathy but not vitamin D deficiency. Diabetes Medicine. 2017;**34**:839-845

[26] Sidawy AN. Diabetic Foot: Lower Extremity Arterial Disease and Limb Salvage. Lippincott Williams & Wilkins; 2006

[27] National Institute for Health and Care Excellence. Diabetic Foot Problems: Prevention and Management [Online]. 2015. Available form: https://www.nice.org.uk/guidance/ng19. [Accessed: September 13, 2018]

[28] Fernández-Torres R, Ruiz-Muñoz M, Pérez-Panero AJ, García-Romero JC, Gónzalez-Sánchez M. Clinician assessment tools for patients with diabetic foot disease: A systematic review. Journal of Clinical Medicine. 2020;**9**(5):1487. DOI: 10.3390/jcm9051487. PMID: 32429068; PMCID: PMC7291260

[29] van Doremalen RFM, van Netten JJ, van Baal JG, Vollenbroek-Hutten MMR, van der Heijden F. Validation of low-cost smartphone-based thermal camera for diabetic foot assessment. Diabetes Research and Clinical Practice.

2019;**149**:132-139. DOI: 10.1016/j.diabres.2019.01.032

[30] Forsythe RO, Hinchliffe RJ. Assessment of foot perfusion in patients with a diabetic foot ulcer. Diabetes/Metabolism Research and Reviews. 2016;**32**:232-238. DOI: 10.1002/dmrr.2756

[31] Schaper NC, Nabuurs-Franssen MH. The diabetic foot: Pathogenesis and clinical evaluation. Seminars in Vascular Medicine. 2002;**2**(2):221-228

[32] Scottish Intercollegiate Guidelines Network. SIGN 116. Management of Diabetes. A National Clinical Guideline. 2010. http://www.sign.ac.uk/pdf/sign116.pdf. [Accessed May 18, 2015]

[33] Diabetic foot problems: prevention and management. London: National Institute for Health and Care Excellence (NICE); 2019 Oct. (NICE Guideline, No. 19.) ISBN-13: 978-1-4731-1387-9

[34] Diabetes UK. Putting feet first. Fast Track for a Foot Attack: Reducing Amputations. 2013. Available from: https://www.slideshare.net/HSCIC/benefits-case-study-diabetes-uk-putting-feet-first-campaign-55929268

[35] Boyko EJ, Ahroni JH, Davignon D, Stensel V, Prigeon RL, Smith DG. Diagnostic utility of the history and physical examination for peripheral vascular disease among patients with diabetes mellitus. Journal of Clinical Epidemiology. 1997;**50**(6):659-668

[36] Suzuki E, Kashiwagi A, Nishio Y, et al. Increased arterial wall stiffness limits flow volume in the lower extremities in type 2 diabetic patients. Diabetes Care. 2001;**24**(12):2107-2114

[37] Lewis JEA, Owens DR. The pulse volume recorder as a measure of peripheral vascular status in people with diabetes mellitus. Diabetes Technology & Therapeutics. 2010;**12**(1):75-80

[38] Ezio F, Giacomo C, Maurizio C, Antonella Q, Vincenzo C, Francesco S. Evaluation of feasibility of ankle pressure and foot oxymetry values for the detection of critical limb ischemia in diabetic patients. Vascular and Endovascular Surgery. 2010;**44**(3):184-189

[39] Cina C, Katsamouris A, Megerman J, et al. Utility of transcutaneous oxygen tension measurements in peripheral arterial occlusive disease. Journal of Vascular Surgery. 1984;**1**(2):362-371

[40] Castronuovo JJ, Adera HM, Smiell JM, Price RM. Skin perfusion pressure measurement is valuable in the diagnosis of critical limb ischemia. YMVA. 1997;**26**(4):629-637. DOI: 10.1016/S0741-5214(97)70062-4

[41] Urabe G, Yamamoto K, Onozuka A, Miyata T, Nagawa H. Skin perfusion pressure is a useful tool for evaluating outcome of ischemic foot ulcers with conservative therapy. Annals of Vascular Diseases. 2009;**2**(1):21-26

[42] Braun JD, Trinidad-Hernandez M, Perry D, Armstrong DG, Mills JL. Early quantitative evaluation of indocyanine green angiography in patients with critical limb ischemia. Journal of Vascular Surgery. 2013;**57**(5):1213-1218

[43] Ludyga T, Kuczmik WB, Kazibudzki M, et al. Ankle-brachial pressure index estimated by laser Doppler in patients suffering from peripheral arterial obstructive disease. Annals of Vascular Surgery. 2007;**21**(4):452-457

[44] Boulton AJM. Late sequelae of diabetic neuropathy. In: AJM B,

editor. Diabetic Neuropathy. Vol. 1997. Lancaster: Marius Press; 1997. pp. 63-76

[45] Mayfield JA, Reiber GE, Sanders LJ, Janisse D, Pogach LM. Preventive foot care in people with diabetes. Diabetes Care. 1998;**21**:2161-2177

[46] Reiber GE, Vileikyte L, Boyko EJ, Del Aguila M, Smith DG, Lavery LA, et al. Causal pathways for incident lower-extremity ulcers in patients with diabetes from two settings. Diabetes Care. 1999;**22**:157-162

[47] Veves A, Murray HJ, Young MJ, Boulton AJM. The risk of foot ulceration in diabetic patients with high foot pressures; a prospective study. Diabetologia. 1992;**35**:660-663

[48] Pham H, Armstrong DG, Harvey C, Harkless LB, Giurini JM, Veves A. Screening techniques to identify people at high risk for diabetic foot ulceration. A prospective multicenter trial. Diabetes Care. 2000;**23**:606-611

[49] Veves A, Sarnow MR, Giurini JM, et al. Differences in joint mobility and foot pressure between black and white diabetic patients. Diabetic Medicine. 1995;**12**:585-589

[50] Frykberg RG, Lavery LA, Pham H, Harvey C, Harkless L, Veves A. Role of neuropathy and high foot pressures in diabetic foot ulceration. Diabetes Care. 1998;**21**:1714-1719

[51] Delbridge L, Perry P, Marr S, et al. Limited joint mobility in the diabetic foot: Relationship to neuropathic ulceration. Diabetic Medicine. 1988;**5**:333-337

[52] Mueller MJ, Diamond JE, Delitto A, Sinacore DR. Insensitivity, limited joint mobility, and plantar ulcers in patients with diabetes mellitus. Physical Therapy. 1989;**69**:453-462

[53] Fitzcharles MA, Duby S, Waddell RW, Banks E, Karsh J. Limitation of joint mobility (cheiroarthropathy) in adult noninsulin-dependent diabetic patients. Annals of the Rheumatic Diseases. 1984;**43**:251-257

[54] Bojsen-Møller F. Anatomy of the forefoot, normal and pathologic. Clinical Orthopaedics and Related Research. 1979;**142**:10-18

[55] Gooding GA, Stess RM, Graf PM, et al. Sonography of the sole of the foot: Evidence for loss of foot pad thickness in diabetes and its relationship to ulceration of the foot. Investigative Radiology. 1986;**21**(1):45-48

[56] Abouaesha F, van Schie CHM, Griffths GD, et al. Plantar tissue thickness is related to peak plantar pressure in the high-risk diabetic foot. Diabetes Care. 2001;**24**(7):1270-1274

[57] Cavanagh PR. Plantar soft tissue thickness during ground contact in walking. Journal of Biomechanics. 1999;**32**(6):623-628

[58] Jan YK, Lung CW, Cuaderes E, et al. Effect of viscoelastic properties of plantar soft tissues on plantar pressures at the first metatarsal head in diabetics with peripheral neuropathy. Physiological Measurement. 2012;**34**(1):53

[59] Hsu CC, Tsai WC, Shau YW, et al. Altered energy dissipation ratio of the plantar soft tissues under the metatarsal heads in patients with type 2 diabetes mellitus: A pilot study. Clinical biomechanics. 2007;**22**(1):67-73

[60] Deschamps K, Matricali GA, Roosen P, et al. Comparison of foot

segmental mobility and coupling during gait between patients with diabetes mellitus with and without neuropathy and adults without diabetes. Clinical biomechanics. 2013;**28**(7):813-819

[61] DiLiberto FE, Tome J, Baumhauer JF, et al. Individual metatarsal and forefoot kinematics during walking in people with diabetes mellitus and peripheral neuropathy. Gait & Posture. 2015;**42**(4):435-441

[62] Cheing GLY, Chau RMW, Kwan RLC, et al. Do the biomechanical properties of the ankle–foot complex influence postural control for people with type 2 diabetes? Clinical Biomechanics. 2013;**28**(1):88-92

[63] Guney AF, Karaman VI, Kafadar IH, et al. Biomechanical properties of Achilles tendon in diabetic vs. non-diabetic patients. Exper Clin Endocrin. Diabetes. 2015;**123**(7):428-432

[64] Caselli A, Pham H, Giurini JM, et al. The forefoot-to-rearfoot plantar pressure ratio is increased in severe diabetic neuropathy and can predict foot ulceration. Diabetes Care. 2002;**25**(6):1066-1071

[65] Guldemond NA, Leffers P, Walenkamp GHIM, et al. Prediction of peak pressure from clinical and radiological measurements in patients with diabetes. BMC Endocrine Disorders. 2008;**8**(1):16

[66] D'ambrogi E, Giacomozzi C, Macellari V, Uccioli L. Abnormal foot function in diabetic patients: The altered onset of windlass mechanism. *Diabetic Medicine*. 2005;**22**(12):1713-1719

[67] Courtemanche R, Teasdale N, Boucher P, et al. Gait problems in diabetic neuropathic patients. *Archives of Physical Medicine and Rehabilitation*. 1996;**77**(9):849-855

[68] Kwon OY, Minor SD, Maluf KS, Mueller MJ. Comparison of muscle activity during walking in subjects with and without diabetic neuropathy. Gait & Posture. 2003;**18**(1):105-113

[69] Craig ME, Duffin AC, Gallego PH, et al. Plantar fascia thickness, a measure of tissue glycation, predicts the development of complications in adolescents with type 1 diabetes. Diabetes Care. 2008;**31**(6):1201-1206

[70] Hazari A, Maiya AG, Shivashankara KN, Monteiro MA, Kumar CS, Rao K, et al. 3D biomechanical analysis of foot in diabetes with and without peripheral neuropathy-a pilot study. Research Journal of Pharmaceutical, Biological and Chemical Sciences. 2016;**7**(3):558-564